KETONE POWER

Superfuel for Optimal Mental Health and Ultimate Physical
Performance

CRISTIAN VLAD ZOT

Table of Contents

Introduction

Since there is too much information out there, many people really don't know who to follow and what to listen to. Information is not important now. What is important is how one is able to manipulate information, how to interpret it and how to use it to achieve greater benefits in their life.

In terms of nutrition and well being there is a lot going on right now. Some say fruits are bad, others say dairy is bad, while others say that consuming too many vegetables is bad. If you would have to listen to all that is said, you would not be able to eat anything.

The paradigm of nutrition will most likely shift to personalized nutrition in the years to come. We are different human beings and "one size to fit them all" should not apply to diet.

Experts and professionals in personal nutrition will have a lot to gain because this industry will explode. The level of personalization will apply to different variables, such as age, physical health, the purpose of a certain nutrition, etc.

Now you may be wondering what this book is all about. I wanted to write it ever since I started seeing amazing result with my ketogenic experiment. This book represents my manifesto to the misleading information that's promoted via the media and through dietary guidelines in terms of nutrition and health. Take it as a point of view (my point of view). Do not take it for granted but conduct your own research and see how it applies to your life.

It is also written as an expression of gratitude to all the wonderful virtual mentors that I had along my journey, such as: Peter Attia, Tim Ferriss, Dr. Stephen Phinney, Dr. Eric Westman, Dr. Jeff Volek, Gary Taubes, Thomas Seyfried, Mark Sisson, Doug McGuff, Dr. Stephen Sinatra, Johnny Bowden, and many other experts from various fields.

Again, I want you to start asking yourself some questions about the type of food that is being promoted to you as healthy and then conduct your own research.

This book is about high-fat-very-low-carbohydrate (ketogenic) nutrition. It follows my personal experience on the subject and it links back to the research in this field. The whole purpose is to help you, the uninitiated reader, to better understand how nutrition has a powerful impact on your well being, on your health, as well as on your mental performance.

Since I'm writing this book for the general public, I will try to use as much non-technical language as possible so that the level of understanding reaches the broader audience.

Special thanks go to my friends who helped me to edit the book and make it more comprehensive. David Hermann, you'd definitely make a professional editor wanna quit his job. Thank you Bill Lagakos, Cornel Paina, and Andrei Tit. Your help is ever appreciated.

31.01.2014   Cristian Vlad Zot

Measurements

Before getting started I'd like to make it easier for you to convert from one unit of measurement to another because I've written this book using the metric system and some of you may be accustomed to the imperial system. Here are the most common units to convert. If there is something you cannot find, just Google: "x" unit metric unit imperial or vice-versa (ex: 1 meter yards, 1 meter inches, 100g ounces, etc.)

Metric	=>	Imperial
1 millimeter [mm]		0.0394 in
1 centimeter [cm]	10 mm	0.3937 in
1 meter [m]	100 cm	1.0936 yd
1 kilometer	1000 m	0.6214 mile
1 milligram [mg]		0.0154 grain
1 gram [g]	1000 mg	0.0353 oz
1 kilogram [kg]	1000 g	2.2046 lb
1 ton [t]	1000 kg	0.9842 long ton
1 Liter [L]		0.264 gal
0 degrees Celsius		32 degrees Fahrenheit
100 degrees Celsius		212 degrees Fahrenheit

Imperial	=>	Metric
1 inch [in]		2.54 cm
1 foot [ft]	12 in	0.3048 m
1 yard [yd]	3 ft	0.9144 m
1 mile	1760 yd	1.6093 km
1 ounce [oz]	437.5 grain	28.35 g
1 pound [lb]	16 oz	0.4536 kg
1 gallon [gal]		3.785 L

Chapter One

When Nothing seems to work, adopt the Uncommon

That evening I jumped onto the scale and boom: 75.6kg. I was far behind the physical goals that I set for myself a few years ago. I felt that I was slowly sliding away from a state that I would like to call "good fitness". It was a Sunday evening of September 2013 and I was at the end of a binging day.

For those of you who don't know what binging is (in the context of dieting) it refers to the day of the week when you allow yourself to eat as much as you can and whatever you want. Some people call it a cheat day. You literally can eat until you throw up. However, the other 6 days of the week, you have to be a monk in terms of nutrition. You "gather" all the cravings throughout the week and you express them in an orgasmic-like form during the binging day. I learned about binging when following Tim Ferriss' Slow Carb Diet [1].

That same Sunday morning my scale was showing 71.8kg. So, I basically added almost 4kg in a single day. That's like ~10 pounds. You may wonder what I'd been eating that particular day. I loaded myself with mountains of refined carbohydrates in various shapes and forms, such as: pizza, cheeseburgers, fries, kebabs, and tons of chocolate. Plus additional water my body demanded to process all those carbohydrates.

Where was I heading? If I kept following that same routine going, things would have gone out of control. And then I had that *Harajaku Moment*. At that particular point in time I had been doing some research (very narrow) on very low carbohydrate diets. I'd been introduced to this study by a short article written by Tim Ferriss on his blog. The article featured Peter Attia and it was on ketosis and athletic performance, a subject that fascinated me tremendously [2].

Before going further, let's jump back in time for a little biographical history of myself.

Throughout my entire life I was a chubby person. I was not obese, but I was overweight, even though I did a lot of exercising. My eating patterns revolved around refined carbohydrates. I ate a lot of pretzels, bread, potatoes, and pizza. That's probably why the load of exercise did not have a big effect on me.

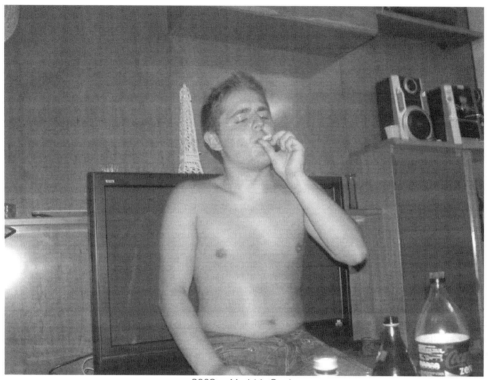
2008 - Madrid, Spain.

However, in March 2010, I had an ear infection that kept me away from my swimming workouts for a couple of weeks. I decided I did not want to give up exercise altogether, so I started doing push-ups and the 8 minute abs workout [3]. I did the exercising routine for about two weeks.

The following month, in April 2010, I started doing something that I never did before. I began jogging. I made a new habit out of this sport. Jogging made me change my eating patterns and another great thing happened. I stopped smoking. I had been a smoker for more than 9 years. And I was only 21 back in 2010.

In terms of eating, I removed a big amount of refined carbohydrates from my diet. The effect was immediate. From the overweight person (~80kg, given that I was 173 cm tall), I got to be a slim person of 67kg. These results had been achieved in ~8 weeks. It was my initial fat-loss.

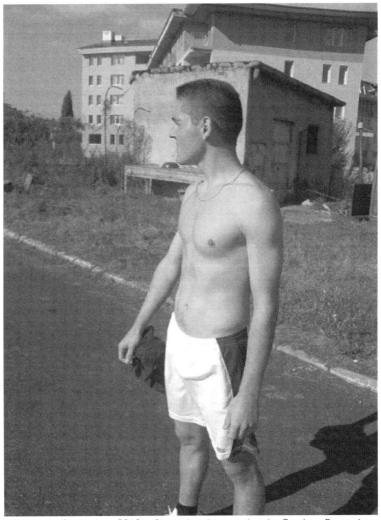
Taken in September 2010, after a jogging session in Oradea, Romania.

I've been reviewing my food logs from back then and I can tell you that I was mostly eating: fruits, whole wheat products, dairy products, peanuts, cheese, tomatoes, cucumbers, and low-fat meats. It may seem that I was still eating a lot of carbohydrates (in the context of a ketogenic diet which is a very low carbohydrate diet), but there were way fewer carbohydrates than I previously consumed. I was loading up on vegetables and fruits mostly.

The average caloric intake was somewhere around 2300 kcals and I was exercising every day. The activities that I was doing were: jogging, kickboxing, indoor exercising, cycling, and soccer.

In the couple of months and years that followed, I maintained the same routine in terms of eating and exercising. 6 days of the week I was eating low-carb (very responsibly) while 7th day was a binging day. Things have changed at the beginning of 2013, when my fitness goals changed.

I wanted to put on some muscle and I was under the impression that I had to eat a lot of protein and do some weight lifting. I thought I could build muscle easily so I added some carbs to my diet as well.

I started weight lifting in January 2013. Up until June the same year I went from 68 to 73 kg. I could not tell if that was fat or muscle. I was not truly satisfied with my results because I measured my arms, legs, waist, shoulders, etc and I did not see significant change, other than my abs getting less visible.

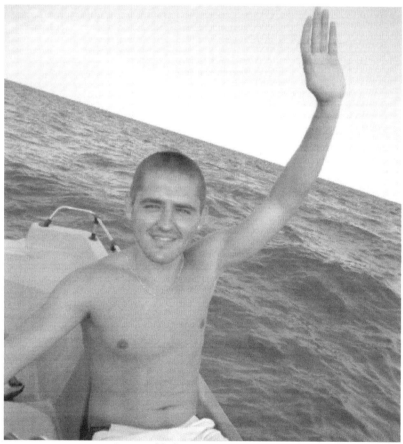
August, 2013 - Black Sea, Romania.

I was always frustrated because I never had the abs I wanted to have, even though I was exercising to exhaustion. And now even those modest abs were becoming less visible.

During that summer of 2013 I also tried the PAGG + Slow Carb Diet Approach of Tim Ferriss, but regretfully I didn't get the results I expected. It may have been probably because I wasn't going as low carb as expected. My binging Sundays were a total feast.

I'll talk more about PAGG in a later chapter.

So, here we are, back in September 2013. I knew that I had to make a drastic change if I wanted to have the six packs that I always dreamed of.

Enter Ketones

The very next week I decided to go all-in with the ketogenic diet. This type of diet requires you to eat more than 60% of the total calories as fat, 30-35% of the total calories as proteins, and 5-10% as carbohydrates. For me it wasn't very difficult to do it because I was already on a low-carb routine.

Whenever you reduce dietary carbohydrates this way (eat less than 30g of carbohydrates/day), your body shifts the metabolism from burning sugar to utilizing fat for fuel. This means that your body adapts to burning fat for energy, instead of sugar (of which the body is deprived of).

*sugar is a carbohydrate. I often use them interchangeably.

I was able to enter ketosis (the metabolic state where your body uses fat for energy) quickly and I stayed in ketosis for the next two months. These were the two greatest months of my life.

Not only that I lost 4.2kg of fat while eating mostly fat, but there were other benefits: more energy throughout the day, better sleep (I slept for 5 hours/night and never felt tired during the day), increased mental sharpness, no hunger, no cravings for sweets and sugary foods, increased physical performance (after keto-adaptation), as well as other health benefits. I actually documented my experiment in a post on my blog [4]. Each of these benefits will be treated in details in the following chapters.

After the experiment ended on December 10, 2013, the results were: 4.2kg of bodyweight lost (which was all fat) and a slightly increase in lean mass. The highest percentage of fat that I lost was from my abdominal area, as it is visible in the DXA scans below (before and after).

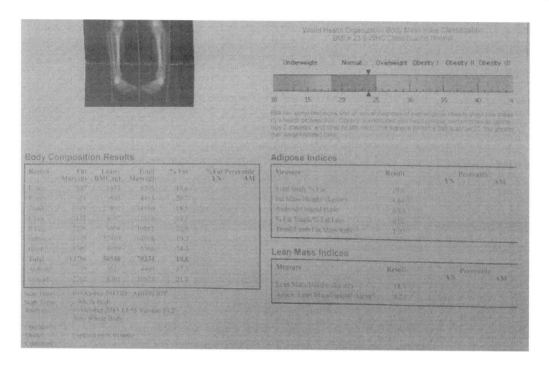

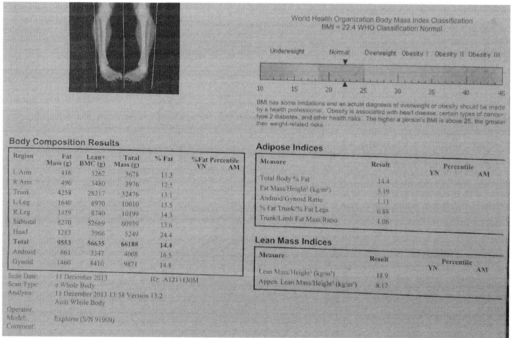

Body Composition Results

Region	Fat Mass (g)	Lean+ BMC (g)	Total Mass (g)	% Fat	%Fat Percentile YN	%Fat Percentile AM
L Arm	416	3262	3678	11.3		
R Arm	496	3480	3976	12.5		
Trunk	4258	28217	32476	13.1		
L Leg	1640	8970	10610	15.5		
R Leg	1459	8740	10199	14.3		
Subtotal	8270	52669	60939	13.6		
Head	1283	3966	5249	24.4		
Total	9553	56635	66188	14.4		
Android	661	3347	4008	16.5		
Gynoid	1460	8410	9871	14.8		

Scan Date: 11 December 2013   ID: A1211130M
Scan Type: e Whole Body
Analysis: 11 December 2013 13:38 Version 13.2
Auto Whole Body
Operator:
Model: Explorer (S/N 91909)
Comment:

Adipose Indices

Measure	Result	Percentile YN	AM
Total Body % Fat	14.4		
Fat Mass/Height² (kg/m²)	3.19		
Android/Gynoid Ratio	1.11		
% Fat Trunk/% Fat Legs	0.88		
Trunk/Limb Fat Mass Ratio	1.06		

Lean Mass Indices

Measure	Result	Percentile YN	AM
Lean Mass/Height² (kg/m²)	18.9		
Appen. Lean Mass/Height² (kg/m²)	8.17		

The full version of the scans: http://cristivlad.com/ketoexperiment

Since I've been learning and experimenting with ketogenic diets and ketosis for the entire period of time between September and December 2013, I started to love everything that had something to do with the concept of high-fat-very-low-carb.

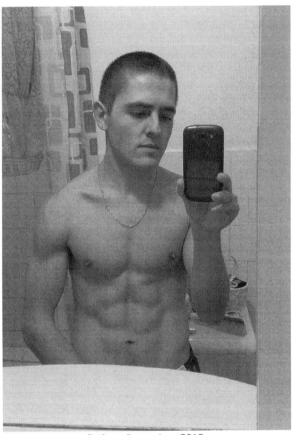
Selfie - December 2013.

I also decided that I was going to stick with maintaining ketosis because it is an extremely pleasant metabolic state and it has a lot of advantages. Besides, I never felt deprived in terms of food and I never felt hungry. Why on earth would I want to start adding back refined carbohydrates to my diet?

If there's one important take-away from this book, that is: reduce your intake of refined carbohydrates.

In the following chapters I will gradually introduce everything that has to do with ketogenic living, how to enter ketosis, what are the benefits and possible drawbacks, what you can eat, how long until you're fully keto-adapted, how much weight you can lose, as well as other important topics, all being backed up by research studies and by my personal experiences.

Chapter Two

Sugar or Fat? A Story of Two Metabolisms

The human body can get the energy it needs for daily expenditure in two primary ways: by metabolizing glucose or by metabolizing fat. Most people nowadays metabolize glucose for energy production. Carbohydrates are the dominant source of calories in the Modern Day World. Glucose is merely the simplest form of Carbohydrate

The body stores glucose in the liver and in the muscles. Whenever it is stored, glucose takes the form of glycogen. However, the body can only store a limited amount of glucose within these deposits and that is approximately 2,000 kcals (calories) [5]. Whatever amount of glucose that you have in your body additionally, that is not used for energy or stored as glycogen, will be turned into fat through the process of lipogenesis [6] and stored into your adipose tissue.

So, if you eat a big pizza, drink some soda, and have a chocolate afterward, your glycogen stores are full because all these foods are carbohydrate rich. And if your energy demands are not big enough, all the carbohydrates that you further consume will go directly into the fat deposits of your body.

Conversely, you can store as much fat as you want on your body (calorically speaking). According to Peter Attia [2], a lean male adult who is approximately 1.80m tall has at least 40,000 kcals stored within his body as body fat. Compare that to the 2,000 kcals that can be stored as glycogen. Things get a bit more complicated when we wish to use body fat for energy production.

Note: *I will mostly use the metric system when referring to units of weight, length, temperature, etc. For conversions to pounds, inches, and other units, just use an online converter or see the beginning of the book.*

A normal person following the standard American diet (which is a high-carbohydrate diet - 60% carbs) will not be able to access most of his fat storage for conversion to energy even with high intensity exercise.

That is why most of the athletes (who are on high-carbohydrate nutrition) running marathons will feel exhausted after depleting their glycogen stores.

The basic idea is that under high-carbohydrate nutrition, one cannot efficiently use body fat for fuel. To do so, one would have to drastically restrict carbohydrate intake. This is because hormonal signaling and enzyme activity are different for these two metabolic pathways. The energy equation may also look different.

Why is that? Who is the culprit?

First of all, it is insulin. Some would like to call it the fat regulating hormone or the guardian of fat [7]. Whenever insulin levels are high (that's when blood glucose levels are increased), both the fat and the excess carbohydrates from food will go straight into the fat storage [6].

Whenever insulin levels are low, your body is able to mobilize fat from fat storage to use it for fuel (energy production). In healthy individuals insulin levels are low when blood sugar (serum glucose) is low. To maintain a low level of blood sugar, you would have to dramatically restrict carbohydrate intake.

Hopefully I haven't lost you so far. Please bear with me and try to understand the moderately technical language that I use because these are important concepts that we will later refer to.

You want to be able to efficiently access your body fat to use it as fuel, instead of using carbohydrates (in their basic form of glucose).

If my blood glucose levels are very low, how would I have the energy to do whatever I do in a particular day? How can I exercise when I need carbohydrates to keep me energized?

It's not easy these days to send a different message that is totally contradictory to the general dogma and to the medical guidelines for proper nutrition. The industry of wellness and sports' nutrition is generating billions every year promoting the same products and the same messages: that you need carbohydrates for energy and for working out efficiently.

However, studies have shown that humans can effectively use fat for fuel and for energy production [8]. From an evolutionary perspective, the human species has been following the same high-fat-low-carb diet for more than 2 million years.

Our ancestors did not have grains and other foods very rich in carbohydrates. They didn't have refined carbohydrates. And they did not have easy access to food whenever they wanted. Getting food was usually a constant struggle.

Grains generally became available ~10,000 years ago. That's a very small period of time compared to 2 million years of human evolution. Many of us are not adapted to process such a huge load of carbohydrates every day. That's why the epidemics of diabetes and obesity have been increasing tremendously in the past 50 years.

Phinney and Volek have conducted a research study [9] in which they measured the athletic performance of 5 cyclists before and after a period of 5 weeks on a very low carbohydrate diet. During the 5 weeks period, the cyclists consumed approximately 20g of carbohydrates/day while the rest of the calories came from fat (mostly) and protein (moderately).

The cyclists did not show decrease in their performance. Rather, they show a dramatic reduction in glucose oxidation (production of energy from glucose), which means they were mostly using fat (either as ketone bodies or fatty acids) for energy production. Bottom line, their performance was not compromised, as the researchers concluded.

How is my mental performance going to change? Everybody knows that the brain is glucose (sugar) dependent.

This is another good question and it has to be addressed from the very beginning. The human brain uses approximately a third of the total daily energy expenditure (TEE). That's somewhere around 600 kcals/day. And since that energy needs to come from glucose, hence carbohydrates, it means you would have to ingest about 150g of carbohydrates every day to meet the energy demands of your brain (1g of carbohydrate yields 4 kcals).

If this were true, then all the people on low and very low carbohydrate diets would be dead. To illustrate, in order for you to be on a ketogenic diet (thus, be in ketosis) you would have to restrict carbohydrate intake to less than 50g/day. Some people must restrict carbohydrates even further, somewhere to < 30g/day.

Studies [11] have shown that the human brain can get its energy from two sources: glucose or ketones (a ketone body is created in the liver from fatty acids). There is no difference in terms of mental performance when your brain runs on BOHB (beta-hydroxibutirate - a ketone body) rather than fat.

More over, studies have shown that BOHB can serve as a more efficient brain fuel compared to glucose. There are fewer oxidative processes within the brain when the major source of fuel is not coming from carbohydrates. Besides, BOHB has neuro-protective properties [10].

Ketogenic (very-low-carbohydrate-high-fat) diets have been used to treat brain disorders such as: Epilepsy, Parkinson's Disease, Alzheimer and others since the beginning of the 20th century.

Rule 1: Restrict Carbohydrates

If you decide that you want to try this out, here are the most important things that you need to know.

Disclaimer

First of all, I do not own a medical degree and I take no responsibility for possible negative implications that this may have on you. Everything that I write here is based on the experiences that I've conducted on my body and also based on the research that I did in this field.
Consult with your medical care practitioner before attempting any modification to your diet.

Think of the ketogenic nutrition as something that you would try out for a moderate to long period of time. You cannot just do it for a couple of days because it will have no effect.

Even though you enter ketosis (the metabolic state where you primarily use fat for energy production) after 2 or 3 days of carbohydrate restriction, it takes at least a couple of weeks until your body is fully keto-adapted (until it has created all the enzymes and mitochondria necessary to support this type of metabolism).

This does not mean that it will take that much longer for you to experience the benefits of ketosis and ketogenic nutrition.

I personally started my ketogenic experiment in late September - the beginning of October 2013. After a couple of days of drastically restricting carbohydrates I was in ketosis. Some people have to go as low as 30g or even 20g, while others can go up to as much as 50g or even 100g of carbohydrates per day. My initial target was < 50g.

I knew I was in ketosis because I had bought some ketone strips that measure urine ketone levels.

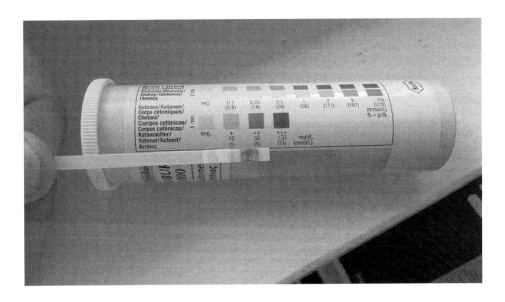

Ketone bodies are produced by your liver when you dramatically cut-off the intake of carbohydrates. These ketone bodies are: acetone, aceto-acetate, and beta-hydroxibutirate. In ketosis, the level of ketones in your body is elevated.

There is also another state when ketone levels are elevated in your body. It's called diabetic ketoacidosis and the level of ketones in your body is several fold increased compared to nutritional ketosis (the one that we go for).

To illustrate, you enter ketosis when ketone levels go above 0.5 mmol/L (either measured in serum or in the urine). It can go up to 3-6 mmol/L depending on the level of exercise and nutrition that you are following. On the other hand, in diabetic ketoacidosis the blood ketones are exceeding 10mmol/L. In ketoacidosis blood glucose level is elevated as well, while in ketosis blood glucose level is normal. Here's a simple and very illustrative graph from Dr. Steve Phinney and Dr. Jeff Volek's book [5] for a better understanding of the topic.

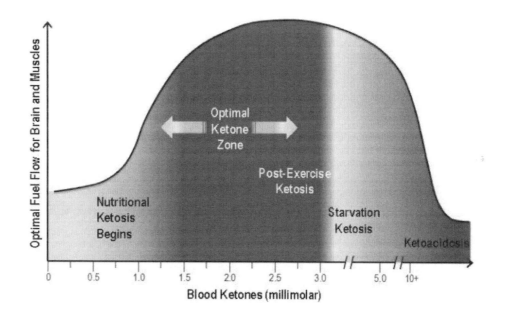

As you restrict your carbohydrate intake, it is only a matter of time until you are in ketosis. There are various ways to measure whether or not you're in this state. You can use urine ketone strips [12] (the same way that I used them) or you can use a blood monitoring system, like the one from Abbot [13]. There are also newer ways of doing it, but they imply higher costs so they will not be discussed here.

When you use the blood ketone measuring system, you have to buy the strips, which are quite expensive ($3-$5 per strip). So, I'd recommend use the urine tests which are somewhere between $10-$20 for a pack of 50 tests.

One of the chapters of the book will address possible foods to consume to maintain ketosis, foods to avoid, as well as certain meal plans that you can follow to support this lifestyle.

So, don't forget that the most important principle for you to know right now (if you want to be in ketosis) is **to restrict carbohydrates to as low as 30g per day**.

The next chapter addresses what happens in your body in the first few weeks of nutritional ketosis. I'll tell you what I've personally been through and I'll outline the potential pitfalls you may want to avoid.

Chapter Three

The Beginning of an Amazing Journey

Keto-adaptation is a process that undergoes for at least a few weeks, a process in which the body completely adapts to using ketones (by-products of fat oxidation in the liver) as the primary source of fuel. It does so by creating all the enzymes and metabolites necessary to facilitate this type of metabolism.

If you've been a high-carb consumer, this process may have some effects on you. Think of it this way: since you're depriving your body from the source of energy it's been used to for so long, how would you expect it to feel and react? Give your body sufficient time and it will gradually adapt.

The most common negative effects of keto-adaptation are: fatigue, headaches, light-headedness, as well as other symptoms. However, many people do not have these experiences while undergoing the process of adaptation. On the contrary, their general state of well-being is improved.

Most of these effects show up because of an imbalance in vitamins and minerals. When first starting a very-low-carb-high-fat lifestyle (or approach) many people will lose a lot of water in the first few days. Your body sheds excess water because it doesn't have to support a big intake of carbohydrates (which need water to be properly processed by the body). However, dehydration is not desired in ketosis and your body does not like that.

Since you do not retain water, your sodium (salt) intake will most likely go down. This is where you have to take action. Phinney and Volek [5] suggest the intake of a few grams of sodium chloride (salt) every day so that the chemical balance in the body is maintained. If you don't want to add additional salt to your food, you can use broth to make up for the excretion of sodium from your body. This should eliminate lightheadedness, headaches, as well as dehydration.

Another possible negative effect that many people report is constipation. This could be due either to the lower water intake, lower fiber intake or, sometimes, because of eating too much cheese. Let me explain.

Since you do not consume large amounts of carbohydrates and since fats are water insoluble, you will most likely not feel thirsty throughout the day. Hence, your water consumption will decrease. This is not okay because your body needs a sufficient amount of water to be able to sustain the balance within. Salt intake combined with drinking fair amounts of water should reduce or eliminate this issue.

Also, fiber intake may also go down on high-fat diets. This is also not okay because fiber facilitates movement within your bowels. Make sure your intake of fiber is between 20-30g/day and make sure it comes from leafy green vegetables, broccoli, kale, or other non-starchy sources. We'll focus on food in later chapters. A good way to mitigate constipate is to consume 1-2 tsps of coconut oil.

If you still experience constipation (even though you shouldn't if you follow the guidelines), try supplementing with psyllium, which is very rich in fiber [18].

I personally experienced this negative effect and I assumed it was because I was consuming way too much cheese (more than 200g/day), not drinking enough water, and not eating enough fiber. I was able to eliminate it by adding psyllium husk into my protein shake, by drinking 3-5 glasses of water throughout the day, and by consuming less cheese.

Back to keto-adaptation and its early history, Phinney [14] has studied the findings of Lt. Friederick Schwatka who did an expedition in 1879-1880 searching for the Royal Navy Franklin crew. The expedition lasted for almost a year (from April 1879 to March 1880) and it had 18 members. They covered more than 3000 miles (by foot) in very cold weather conditions. Most of their food supply consisted of walrus blubber and the meat from the animals they hunted.

Schwatka recorded personal notes throughout the entire expedition. Here's a transcript that was taken from Phinney's [14]:

"When first thrown wholly upon a diet of reindeer meat, it seems inadequate to properly nourish the system, and there is an apparent weakness and inability to perform severe exertive fatiguing journeys. But this soon passes away in the course of two or three weeks."

However, one can minimize the side effects of carbohydrate deprivation during keto-adaptation. The wise strategy in this case would be to reduce carbohydrate progressively and not all at once. This means that you can go the first 1 or 2 weeks on a moderately low carbohydrate diet, where you restrict carbohydrates to less than 150g/day, given that you were previously consuming more than 400-500 grams of carbohydrates per day. After these two weeks, you can try and restrict carbohydrates to less than 30g/day.

Overall, my keto-adaptation process was pleasant because I was coming from a period of low-carbohydrate intake (with carbohydrate cycling once per week). So, I was probably ingesting 100-150g/carbohydrates/day for up to two months prior to entering ketosis.

My Slow-Carb Approach

At the beginning of the summer of 2013 I started following Tim Ferriss' Slow Carb Diet [1].

1. My breakfast:

100g salted peanuts
1 apple
150g yoghurt
50g of whole grain biscuits

This wasn't exactly very low carb, but it was lower than my previous diet had been.

2. My lunch (if you can call it lunch):

2 protein bars - 120g
50g of whole grain biscuits
and, usually a big unsweetened lemonade or squeezed grapefruit.

3. My dinner:

150g mixed vegetables (usually Mexican mix)
150g of chicken breast or 3 eggs
150g cabbage salad with dressing (oil, vinegar, salt, pepper).

Let's break it down in terms of carbohydrates:

100g salted peanuts = 6g net carbs
1 apple = 12g net carbs
150g yoghurt = 6g net carbs
50g of whole grain biscuits = 30g net carbs
2 protein bars - 120g = 50g net carbs
50g of whole grain biscuits = 30g net carbs
big unsweetened lemonade or squeezed grapefruit with it = 0 carbs
150g mixed vegetables (usually Mexican mix) = 6 net carbs
150g of chicken breast or 3 eggs = 0 net carbs
150g cabbage salad with dressing (oil, vinegar, salt, pepper). = 6 net carbs

Total net carbs = 146g

My Ketogenic Approach

When I started the ketogenic experiment [4], my menu was radically altered. Here's the breakdown, in approximate terms:

1. Breakfast

100g oil roasted peanuts, with salt
50g of cheese

2. Lunch (or snack #1)

Salad:

1 avocado ~ 100g
50g curd or pot cheese (which is a type of unsalted cheese)

1/2 squeezed lemon
1 tea spoon of stevia (sweetener)

and

50g low carbohydrate protein bar

3. Dinner

150g fat meat (steak)
100g broccoli, cooked in butter (or kale, or Brussels Sprouts, or some other leafy greens)
20-30g bacon
3-4 olives
30g cheese

4. Second snack (this was and still is extremely rewarding to me)

50g dark chocolate
2-3g goji berries
2-3 teaspoons of peanut butter
30-50g cheese

Again, let's break it down in terms of carbs:

100g oil roasted peanuts, with salt = 6g net carbs
50g of cheese = 0.5g net carbs
1 avocado ~ 100g = 1.5g net carbs
50g curd (which is a type of unsalted cheese) = 2g net carb
1/2 squeezed lemon = 0 net carbs
1 tea spoon of stevia (sweetener) = 0 net carbs
50g low carbohydrate protein bar = 15g net carbs
150g fat meat (steak) = 0 net carbs
100g broccoli cooked in butter (or kale, or Brussels Sprouts, or some other leafy greens) = 4g net carbs
20-30g bacon = 0 net carbs
3-4 olives = < 1g net carbs
30g cheese = < 1g net carbs
50g dark chocolate = 8g net carbs

2-3g goji berries = 1g net carbs
2-3 teaspoons of peanut butter = 2g net carbs
30-50g cheese = 1g net carbs

Total Net Carbs = 43g

During my workout days, I also had a whey isolate protein shake. However, carbohydrate intake was minimal because 1 serving consisted of 1.5g of net carbohydrates.

Net Carbs

Throughout the entire book I will speak in terms of net carbohydrates because most of the fibers are not digestible. Phinney and Volek [5] speak in terms of total carbohydrates but their limit on daily intake is less than 50g (because they include fiber in Total Carbohydrate).

On the other hand, Lyle McDonald [15] refers to net carbohydrates and he recommends a daily intake of 25 to 50g as a good place to start a ketogenic diet.

We will stick to 30g or less of net carbohydrates per day. So:

Net Carbohydrates = Total Carbohydrates - Fibers

Some product labels display *Glucides* instead of *Total Carbohydrates*. This creates a lot of confusion. American labels show both total carbohydrates and fiber so you can do the math by yourself. Some European labels show only total carbohydrates or glucides (which are practically the net carbohydrates) and they do not display the fiber content, while other products show both total carbohydrates and fiber and let you do the math.

I know you may be very confused at this moment, but here's something that will help you sort through the confusion. This is a link to the National Nutrient Database for Standard Reference from U.S.D.A.:

http://ndb.nal.usda.gov/ndb/search/list

Just enter whatever food or product you want to know the amount of net carbohydrates for and subtract *Fiber* from *Total Carbohydrate* to get the net carbs.

To illustrate: You want to know the content of net carbohydrate in oil roasted peanuts (with salt). You just enter "oil roasted peanuts" in the search box and scroll down to "16089, Peanuts, all types, oil-roasted, with salt". After you click on the item, you'll see that:

Carbohydrate, by difference	15.26g
Fiber, total dietary	9.4g

You will get the net carbohydrate by subtracting 9.4 from 15.26. The result is 5.86g of net carbohydrate per 100g of product.

I am sure that you will do this for a while until you know how many net carbohydrates are in the foods you consume. But once you are aware of some values, you'll just know them by heart.

What about calories?

You may notice that I have not referred to calories so far. Most of the diets that we are familiar with focus on restricting calories; they are low calorie diets. Conversely, when you follow a ketogenic (very low carbohydrate diet) the only thing that matters to you is the amount of carbohydrates you ingest. And it is not because of the amount of calories, but because "a calorie is not always a calorie". Let me explain :)

Calories from carbohydrates are different than calories from fat. They trigger different hormonal signaling. Besides, the combination of macronutrients can also stimulate hormones in a different ways. I'm not saying that you should eat 8000kcals while following a ketogenic diet. Try it if you want. You'll do it for a day or two, but then you naturally reduce calories.

If I went on a hunger strike, I would be driven mad with cravings while consuming 1,500kcal of a low calorie high carbohydrate diet. Conversely, I could easily live and be satisfied eating 1,500kcal on a high-fat diet. This is one of the benefits of being keto-adapted.

There are studies showing that a calorie from fat is not the same as a calorie from carbohydrates. Another important thing to know is that the energy equation is different when on different diets. Mostly importantly the "calories-out" (aka the energy burned) is different.

In his book *Good Calories, Bad Calories,* Gary Taubes explains why calories do not matter in the context of low-carb-high-fat diets [16]. He explains the metabolic shift that occurs when a person starts to follow such a diet results in different energy expenditure by the body compared to moderate and high-carbohydrate diets that most people follow.

Ok. Let me be more explicit and explain it again. The total energy expenditure (how many kcals your body consumes per day) is different if you eat 2000 kcals in the context of a high-carb diet than if you eat 2000 kcals in the context of a high-fat very low carbohydrate (ketogenic) diet. The latter will result in more energy expenditure.

The metabolic processes of a person following a ketogenic diet as well as the hormonal implications of these processes are different compared to the metabolic processes of someone following a high-carb diet. You are basically using more energy and burning more calories when you are on a ketogenic diet. Even at rest your body uses more energy if it is adapted to burning fat as the primary source of fuel.

Peter Attia and several other researchers conducted an experiment [2] inside a metabolic chamber. This is a type of chamber that can monitor all the exchanges of energy that take place between the body and the environment for the purpose of determining the exact amount of energy a body consumes in a day.

During this experiment, Peter was locked inside the metabolic chamber for several days, his food intake was calculated precisely, he had a stationary bike on which he exercised twice a day. He also did plyometric exercises after the cardio sessions (riding the bike). Everything was being monitored. They even monitored his energy expenditure (calories burned/minute) while he was asleep.

His food intake consisted of 2970 kcals, out of which 78.8% was fat, 17.5% was protein, while 3.5% came from carbohydrates.

What they found out was extremely interesting because they have noticed that during resting periods Peter's energy expenditure (or the resting metabolic rate) was 20% higher than predicted. This basically means that at rest (when no physical activity was involved) Peter consumed 20% more calories compared to what was predicted.

This "predicted" is the resting metabolic rate that has been observed in people following a regular high-carbohydrate diet. So, when you are on ketogenic nutrition you use more energy/unit of time even when resting compared to people on high-carb nutrition. This is one thing for which calories don't matter.

Nevertheless, this is a one person experiment (n=1) and it should be taken as such. I want to highlight that each of us are different and that several experiments should be made on higher sample sizes (more subjects) to draw a stronger conclusion.

Now, let's say that you have a 2,500 kcals ketogenic daily menu that would fit your daily energy expenditure in the context of moderate exercising (3-4 times/week).

At least 60% of the 2,500 kcals needs to come from fat. That is 1,500 kcals just from fat. Since 1g of fat is 9kcals, it means you would have to consume ~170g of fat, which (if you ask me) is very satiating.

Another 35% of the 2,500 kcals will come from protein. That is 875 kcals from protein. Since 1g of protein yields 4 kcals, it means you would have to consume ~220g of proteins, which is also very satiating.

The rest of 5% of the 2,500 kcals will come from carbohydrates. That translates to 125 kcals coming from carbohydrates which yield 4 kcals per gram (same as protein). This means you would have to consume ~32g of carbohydrates.

You may be wondering what all these numbers mean and how you can turn them into actual food. Here's how.

100g of fatty meat can have 20-25g of protein and 20-30g of fat. It has 0 carbohydrates. This means you could eat 500g of this type of meat and you still haven't reached your recommended daily intake of protein (~120g) and fat (~170g) if you're a big-buff male.

100g of cooked broccoli can have: ~4g of net carbs, ~2g of protein and 0 fat. If you eat 800g of cooked broccoli/day you would just reach your daily carb intake (~32g). That's almost a kg of broccoli. Who on earth could eat that much + the 500g of meat from above?

These are all exaggerations made with the purpose of giving you a sense of how this kind of nutrition can be approximated in terms of the foods you can eat. It is up to the individual to diversify the diet so that more nutrient dense foods, as well as vitamins and minerals are present in it. There will be a chapter dedicated to foods that you can eat, foods that you can't, as well as a list of possible dishes and menus for ketogenic nutrition.

How did I do it?

Remember the menu that I had when I started ketosis? Let's see how it looks like in terms of calories and macronutrient breakdown:

100g oil roasted peanuts, with salt
6g net carbs   25g protein   50g fat   ~627 kcals

50g of cheese
0.5g net carbs   12g protein   13g fat   ~163 kcals

1 avocado ~ 100g
1.5g net carbs   2g protein   20g fat   ~160 kcals

50g curd or pot cheese (which is a type of unsalted cheese)
2g net carbs   12g protein   8g fat   ~130 kcals

1/2 squeezed lemon
0 net carbs   insignificant   insignificant   insignificant

1 tea spoon of stevia (sweetener)
0 net carbs   insignificant   insignificant   insignificant

50g low carbohydrate protein bar
15g net carbs   12g protein   9g fat   ~190 kcals

150g fat meat (steak)
0 net carbs   35g protein   35g fat   ~430 kcals

100g broccoli cooked in butter (or kale, or Brussels sprouts, or some other leafy greens)
4g net carbs   2g protein   0g fat   ~32 kcals

20-30g bacon
0 net carbs   4g protein   7g fat   ~80 kcals

3-4 olives
< 1g net carbs   insignificant   3g fat   ~30 kcals

30g cheese
< 1g net carbs   8g protein   9g fat   ~105 kcals

50g dark chocolate
8g net carbs   4g protein   25g fat   300 kcals

2-3g goji berries
1g net carbs   insignificant   insignificant   ~10 kcals

2-3 teaspoons of peanut butter
2g net carbs   2g protein   8g fat   ~90 kcals

30-50g cheese
1g net carbs   8g protein   9g fat   ~105 kcals

Total Calories: 2452 kcals
Net carbs: 43g
Protein: 126g
Fat: 196g

Calories from fat: 196 x 9 = 1764 kcals = 71.9%
Calories from protein: 126 x 4 = 504 kcals = 20.5%
Calories from carbs: 43 x 4 = 172 kcals = ~7%

Again, for the sake of better understanding the numbers:

1 oz = ~28g

These are all approximate values. The exact values are not very different from these values. Scrolling through my food logs shows me that the first few weeks in ketosis I actually consumed approximately 3,000 kcals, maintaining the same proportions of macronutrients.

The daily menu that I had may not be relevant or appropriate to many keto dieters. Most of them eat bacon, eggs, and some salad for breakfast. I personally love peanuts and I've been eating them for 4 years now (regularly). It's also convenient for me because I don't have to cook once I get up.

As I entered ketosis, I also dramatically decreased exercise because I was mostly focusing on building traffic for my blog. I was doing 2 workouts (at max) per week. And in those first few weeks I lost approximately 2.5kg of bodyweight, while increasing caloric count and fat intake. Most of this bodyweight lost was probably water.

Up until entering ketosis, I was eating approximately 2000-2200 kcals/day and I was exercising for 6 days a week. I was not able to maintain a stable weight.

The key take away is that the only reason to know how many calories you are ingesting is to make sure that you're eating at least 60% of the total calories as fat, 30-35% at most as protein, and the rest of 5-10% as carbohydrates. For me 70-75% fat, 20% protein, and 5-10% carbohydrates works best so far.

How long does it take to get into ketosis?

Let's assume that it's Sunday evening and you want to shift to ketogenic nutrition starting tomorrow morning. Let's also assume that your glycogen stores are full (which means that your muscles and your liver have ~2000kcals stored as carbohydrates).

To enter ketosis you have to deplete this storage. You do that by dramatically reducing the amount of carbohydrates you ingest.

Remember that the resting metabolic rate for a normal-weight adult male is ~2000-2500kcals while for a normal-weight adult female is ~1600-1900kcals. The resting metabolic rate is the amount of energy that your body consumes over a day to keep you alive. If you were watching TV all day long, that's the amount of energy your body would require.

Let's say you are an active normal-weight adult male and burn approximately 2600-2800kcals/day. Since you ingest a very small amount of carbohydrates, you should be able to enter ketosis in 1-2 days.

However, this is only theoretical. Insulin resistant and obese people, for example, would require more than that. But, in a few days as your body does not have glucose to create energy from, it will start oxidizing fat and creating ketone bodies (acetone, aceto-acetate, and beta-hydroxibutirate) to derive energy from.

Some people have reported to me that they use "fat-fast" or total fast to get into ketosis faster. Others increase their caffeine intake. Others use both strategies. While there may be supporting studies [17] to show that higher-doses of caffeine have an effect on fat oxidation, I did not use any of these techniques, which is why I cannot recommend them. I just wanted to make you aware that if you are really eager to enter ketosis, there may be some ways to cut corners.

How do you measure it?

What I did was to reduce carbohydrate intake to less than 50g/day (I didn't initially go as low as 30g/day) and then after a couple of days my urine ketone tests [12] arrived. I measured urine ketone levels and I was somewhere between 2-3 mmol/L. You can either use the strips [12] or the blood monitoring system [13].

Remember, your actual target is 0.5 - 5 mmol/L. It is okay if you start measuring ketone levels with the strips because they are cheaper. However, as you get keto-adapted they may not be so accurate. Let me explain why this happens.

In the initial phases of ketosis the body starts producing many ketones and some of them (acetoacetate -AcAc- and beta-hydroxibutirate -BOHB-) are excreted through urine. Hence you can use the urine strips. These strips are designed to detect the levels of AcAc.

Phinney and Volek [5] explain that as adaptation proceeds for a couple of weeks, the body is focused on using BOHB for energy. This explains why the production and excretion of AcAc may decrease. Hence, the urine tests may show lower or no traces of ketones in the urine, but this does not mean that the body is not in ketosis.

It simply means that if you really want to know the levels of ketones inside your body, you have to use the blood monitoring system [13] which measures the values of serum BOHB. These are more relevant. After 4 months in ketosis, I can still use the strips but they are less relevant compared to the first few weeks when they always turned to dark pink immediately.

Now What?

Once you know you are in ketosis, you should define your strategy to maintain this state. That is not difficult. Remember the core concepts:

-drastically reduce carbs to 5-10% of total calories,
-increase fat to more than 60% of total calories, while the rest of
-30-35% should be protein.

Within this range of macro-nutrients you have tons of options to design your meals. It's up to your level of creativity and the time you have to spare in the kitchen and experiment.

To know you're doing the right thing, try measuring ketone levels for the first few days up to 1 or 2 weeks. You will notice when these levels tend to be higher, when they are reduced, how they are after a workout, etc. After you have a bigger picture about this, you will most likely stop measuring them, or you will only do it once in a while just to make sure you're on the right track.

In the next chapter we'll see how the body adapts to these metabolic changes and I will tell you more about the benefits that I've experienced as I got keto-adapted.

Chapter Four

I don't want to get out of Ketosis

Weight Loss, Hunger Regulation and No-Cravings Policy

I know this is the part that many of you have been waiting for, so let's get to the nitty gritty of fat loss. This is probably the first and most important reason why many folks consider going on a high-fat-low-carb diet. It's been proven to be very efficient in decreasing the adipose tissue as it uses it for energy production.

There are many studies [19] [20] [21] that show the efficacy of a ketogenic approach to weight loss. Some of these studies followed patients for more than 12 months [19] under this protocol. The researchers have also found a very high rate of compliance with the diet (many of the subjects stick to the research until it ends) compared to lower compliance when subjects have to follow a high-carb hypocaloric diet (low-calorie). Other studies [21] show improved metabolic parameters and higher weight loss in obese children and adolescents on a ketogenic diet compared to a hypocaloric diet.

The first few days of ketosis leads to a few pounds of weight loss which is mostly attributed to water. Subjects lose water because the amount of carbohydrates they eat is substantially lower and their body does not need to retain water to be able to efficiently process these carbohydrates.

Often times this is the reason many people experience headaches and accelerated heart rates (tachycardia). Since they eliminate a lot of water, they tend not to drink enough to make up for the loss (because they are not thirsty), therefore the body gets dehydrated. I'm reminding you that a solution to this problem is to increase sodium (salt) intake.

A few grams of sodium are sufficient and it will lead to a better retention of water by the body. It will also make up for the excretion of Sodium and Potassium from the body which causes a mineral imbalance (often leads to lightheadedness and headaches).

During my experiment I lost ~3kg in the first two weeks of ketosis (I went from 73kg to 70kg). After those two weeks, the process of weight-loss became slower but it was constant.

So, after the initial water loss you will notice a decrease in weight loss, which is normal. You do not have to panic because you still lose fat, but at a slower rate. Let me explain:

Let's say you are two weeks in ketosis and your well formulated ketogenic diet [5] has decreased your hunger and cravings. This means that you will actually eat less from a caloric perspective and feel satisfied. You will create a caloric deficit and this will make your body start using its own adipose tissue to generate the energy it needs.

Two hormones, grehlin and leptin, are responsible for hunger and appetite control, and are influenced by the concentration of insulin in the body (among others). According to Klok et al. [27], leptin mediates long-term energy balance regulation and it suppresses food intake, while ghrelin acts over the short-term and it plays an important role on meal initiation.

High-insulin levels promote fat accumulation and do not allow fat mobilization from adipocytes. The reason is simple. Fat is mobilized from the fat tissue when the body needs energy and it is running low on glucose. However, this is not the case when insulin levels are high. The fat from adipocytes is released when LPL (lipoprotein lipase - an enzyme) is inhibited. LPL signaling (activation) is influenced by insulin levels [29].

Another study [28] began by alluding to the fact that diet-induced weight loss brings changes within the body which have an impact on appetite and encourage weight gain. Their objective was to determine whether or not ketogenic diets suppress appetite in diet-induced weight loss.

To better understand this: after losing weight through diet, ghrelin levels increase and this stimulates appetite and the subjects gain back all the weight that was lost + interest (aka the yoyo effect). In this case [28] the researchers wanted to determine if the same thing happens with ketogenic diets. They did the experiment on 50 overweight subjects. These participants followed an eight week very low calorie ketogenic diet and then 2 weeks following a re-feeding diet.

According to the researchers [28], "when participants were ketotic, the weight loss induced increase in ghrelin was suppressed" while leptin levels decreased as well. So when losing weight via ketogenic diets, these appetite regulating hormones are not stimulated in the same way they are when subjects follow a normal low-calorie weight loss diet. Now, let's see a specific example on how weight (fat) is lost through a ketogenic diet.

Assume that you are a slightly overweight male who is moderately active (3-4 workouts/week). Assume that your total daily energy expenditure is 2600kcals and you eat 2000kcals (65% fat, 30% protein, and 5% carbs). This means that you have a caloric deficit of 600kcals/day. This means that your body needs to use 600kcals from its own energy stores to make up for the deficit. And since there is insignificant carbohydrate storage, your body will use 600kcals from your adipose tissue. Protein is not stored within the body.

We know from previous chapters that 1g of fat = 9kcals. Thus 600kcals is approximately 67g of fat. So you will burn 67g of your own fat in this scenario. Remember that this is a rough approximate, but I just wanted to give you an insight as to what fat loss can potentially mean.

Conversely, if you are following a high-carb diet, it is very difficult for you to burn this amount of fat even under the most stressful conditions (ex: marathons) because your body mostly utilizes glucose for energy.

67g probably seems insignificant and may not be visible on a scale. But if this happens every day for a week (for example) you'll lose 450g (more than 1 pound) of fat. Multiply it by 4 and you have lost 1.8kg of fat/month. This is a big achievement if it's all fat. You can burn even bigger amounts of fat/day as long as you increase your caloric deficit by either exercising or by eating less. Also, remember that I told you that your body uses more energy/minute compared to carbohydrate dependent metabolism. This significantly alters to the whole equation of weight loss.

I personally increased my caloric intake for the first few weeks of ketosis (~3000kcals/day) and I still experienced weight loss. But as I became adapted to utilizing fat my hunger dropped significantly and I naturally started eating less. Right now I'm mostly eating 2200-2500kcals/day and sometimes I need to overeat so that I won't lose more fat.

Bottom line is: once you start losing fat, you will lose it until your body reaches its normal size [5].

Sky-rocket Energy Levels

I am talking a lot about the first few days of a ketogenic diet because this is the point where most of the individuals trying ketosis (for the first time) will quit. Coming from a high-carbohydrate intake background, in the first days of ketosis one can experience several negative effects that I've previously mentioned (headaches, light-headedness, low-energy levels, etc). This is normal because like any change process, it will take a while for your body to adapt to utilizing fat as a primary source of energy.

One can experience lower energy levels because of the low carbohydrate intake and because carbohydrates were formerly the body's most important source of fuel. In these first few days the body is not adapted to primarily oxidizing fat, which explains the negative effects.

But things change if you're able to get over these first few days. As time passes, your body becomes more efficient in burning fat and you start feeling much better. The energy levels start increasing and when you're fully adapted you are at the point in which these energy levels are elevated and they remain constant throughout the day. Let's get to the bottom of it.

I will not dive deep into bio-chemistry and metabolism even though this would be brain porn for many of the geeks. I'll try to explain it as simply as possible and point out some references if you consider yourself a geek.

ATP (adenosine-tri-phosphate) is called the energy currency of the human body. Metabolizing one molecule of glucose will give you a net of 34-38 (the actual number is very debatable) ATPs.

Conversely, metabolizing one molecule of a 16 carbon fatty acid (like Palmitic Acid) will give you a net of 129 ATPs. This means that fatty acid oxidation (or beta-oxidation) can give you over 3 times more energy than metabolizing a molecule of glucose [22] [23]. Also, there is lower oxidative stress (and less inflammation) when your body is powered by ketones [24].

When I was on a high-carbohydrate diet and even when I was on a moderate to low carbohydrate diet (~150g of carbohydrates/day), I did not have decent energy levels. There were times during the day when I felt very tired. Almost every day at approximately one hour after lunch, I just wanted to leave everything and hit the bed.

Working from home allowed me to do so. I experimented with power naps for several months in 2013. These power naps represented my weapons to eliminate the fatigue I felt after eating lunch. They also boosted my mental clarity. Power napping requires 20-30 minutes of sleep during the day. They were very effective for me.

In that period of time, my last meal of the day was at 6 P.M. This raised another problem. I felt tired and wanted to hit the bed for a power nap at 7 P.M. And I often did it. It was kind of crazy.

The craziest period was when I was waking up at 5 A.M., had breakfast at 7 A.M. and then needed a power nap from 7:30 to 8:00 A.M. Most of the people cannot do this if they work for a company. And I think it is very uncomfortable and un-productive to feel extremely tired after eating.

I also had issues waking up in the morning. Sometimes I hit the snooze button of my phone for 2-3 times each 10 minutes before I was able to get out of the bed. This happens because your body uses energy during night-time and since you are on high-carb nutrition your body tends to run low on energy as you wake up in the morning.

So, you can sleep to preserve energy or get a boost in energy through a rich breakfast (orange juice, toast, cereal, and other carbohydrate sources). This tends to create a vicious cycle which will be further discussed in the chapter dedicated to food choices.

Conversely, when you are on a ketogenic diet and your body runs on fat as its primary source of fuel, these things do not happen. It is primarily because your body always has a readily available energy supply. If it is not taken from food, it is taken from your own body fat storage.

As I began to keto-adapt, I started to not feel tired in the morning. I was able to quickly get out of bed. What I also noticed is that I did not require too much sleep and I suspect that the lower oxidative stress + the efficient use of fuel are the reasons I need less sleep by being keto-adapted.

Probably the best thing that happened was the constant flow of energy throughout the day. From the minute I wake up (currently at 7 A.M.) to the minute I go to sleep (currently at 2 A.M.) I never feel tired. I always have high levels of energy, even when I workout (either gym or kickboxing). The after-meal tiredness is gone. I find all these energy-related benefits extremely rewarding because they give me 19 hours per day of increased productivity. This means that I sleep for roughly 5 hours a night and I feel great.

Another positive point is the quality of sleep. I fall asleep within the first five minutes of hitting the bed. I never had problems sleeping before, but when I was on high-carb nutrition there were some times when I couldn't sleep. For example, when I was too tired or when I expected an important event the next day. This has not happened in ketosis so far.

Here's a particular example that can illustrate my experience with energy levels and sleep deprivation in ketosis.

I recently traveled to Thailand for a two-week vacation. My flight should have totaled 28 hours, but it actually lasted twice than that (~52 hours). I was three months in ketosis at that time.

So, I had to travel from Romania to Thailand. It was Tuesday afternoon and I went by minibus from Oradea in Romania to Budapest in Hungary to catch my first flight.

I left Oradea at ~ 2 P.M. on Tuesday and I arrived in Budapest 3 hours later. My flight from Budapest to Moscow was at 11:35 P.M. that same evening. I arrived in Moscow at ~5:30 A.M. (local time) on Wednesday and I wasn't able to sleep during the trip. Probably because it was my first flight.

I had a long connection in Moscow's Sheremetyevo International Airport. My flight from Moscow, Russia to Phuket, Thailand was scheduled for Wednesday evening at 9:45 P.M. So I had to stay in the airport for almost an entire day. There was an area on the floor between two terminals where you could lay down and possibly catch some sleep (if you can ignore all the noise in the airport). I think I was able to sleep for 1 - 1:30 hours on that floor. I could not care less about people passing by and staring at me like I was some sort of freak.

To make things worse, the flight was delayed from 9:45 P.M. to 3:30 A.M. on Thursday. I was extremely irritated when I heard the news, but I was far from feeling tired. Those hours had passed and we finally embarked for the flight which lasted 8 hours and 30 minutes. I was able to sleep for 4 hours in the airplane.

We got in Phuket, Thailand on Thursday at 4:30 P.M local time. It was two days later. So, I left home on Tuesday afternoon and arrived in Thailand on Thursday afternoon. I did not feel I was tired and what's more is that:

I got to my hotel 1 hour later and a friend (who I met over the Internet) came to see me. I quickly unpacked, took a shower, and left with his motorcycle to arrive downtown. It was like 8:30 P.M. on Thursday. We had some drinks (obviously I had low-carb alcohol) and partied up until in the A.M. on Friday. I got back to the hotel and went to sleep at ~4:30 A.M. on Friday. I slept until noon and I didn't feel tired when I woke up.

It hit me as I got back home. I was astonished because I realized that I didn't get a decent sleep for almost three days and I didn't feel sick or tired. It was even more interesting as I correlated this experience with other trips that I did.

For example, last year I went to Crete, a Greek Island. We took the bus thinking that it would be the best alternative since it's cheaper. The major drawback is that it lasted for two freakin' days. I was low-carb back then (150g/day of carbohydrates).

Even so, throughout the whole trip I felt tired and irritated and I was constantly shifting from sleeping states to wakened states since most of the time was spent in the bus. I also had to have a 5-hours sleep when I arrived in Crete. So, there was a huge difference between the two experiences.

Enhanced Mental Focus

I've been talking to a lot of people about the benefits that very-low-carbohydrate nutrition brings to our lives. A common and widely noticed benefit is better mental performance. Let's see what scientific proof we can bring to it (confirmation bias for the win).

When your brain's primary fuel comes from carbohydrates, you constantly need to supply it with this macro-nutrient. That is why individuals who are glucose dependent and feel hungry, often times feel that their mind is foggy and that they cannot think coherently.

That's why if your nutrition is high in carbohydrates and you feel hungry at noon, that hunger can be all that you think of because it is well known that carbohydrates stimulate appetite [26]. Your mental output will most likely decrease.

You enter a vicious circle because if your lunch is high in carbohydrates, it will lead to a spike in insulin levels that will reduce blood glucose. However, when insulin has achieved its target of lowering glucose levels, your body will notice that it runs low on sugar and it will make you feel hungry again.

Sadly, it's only been two hours since lunch and you feel you could have dinner already.

Your brain is the major consumer of glucose in your body. This is something that everyone agrees upon. But the scientific community promoting the very-low-carb-high-fat nutrition will add that: Your brain is the major glucose consumer in your body in the context of high-carbohydrate nutrition. It needs ~600kcals/day. Now, let's see things from a ketogenic perspective.

When you restrict carbohydrates to less than 30g/day, let's assume that your brain will get the entire amount. This translates to 120kcals. What about the rest of energy that it requires to run efficiently? What about the rest of ~480kcals? Well, that energy comes mainly from ketone bodies.

Guzman and Blazquez [10] report that ketone bodies provide a significant contribution to energy production in the brain when glucose is scarce. They have also been shown to have neuroprotective effects. This is also probably credited to the fact that ketogenic diets produce lower oxidative stress throughout the body [26].

To re-emphasize, once you are keto-adapted your body does not run out of fuel. I have previously mentioned that even lean male adults have at least ~40,000kcals stored as fat in their bodies. So, whenever you have used all the energy that came from the food that you've eaten, your body will utilize its rich fat reserves and will use them to produce the fuel it needs. Phinney [5] likes to call ketone bodies "the high-octane fuel that can power our brains".

I think there are many advantages that our brains can experience while running mostly on fat derived energy. First of all, there is the mental clarity and sharp focus throughout the entire day. Second of all, there is a much higher degree of control of emotional states. I've personally noticed that I am better able to control my anger (I don't get angry as often as before). Maybe this is just my biased thinking, but I feel more stable emotionally when running on ketogenic nutrition.

Other people have told me that their anxieties have been reduced ever since they started following a ketogenic diet, while others say that their depression has been reduced or even disappeared. I also find very comforting that I always have the energy available for my brain to run at greater efficiency and that I do not have to charge myself with high-carbohydrate foods every couple of hours just to feel mentally potent.

A Poll On Facebook Groups

While brainstorming for an article a few weeks ago, I posted the same question on various Facebook groups because I wanted to know what people are reporting in terms of the benefits they experience with ketogenic nutrition. Here's what I found. You know what, I'm just gonna post their answers, and hide their names.

B.T. says *"My asthma symptoms really decreased. I rarely have to use my medication now. My insomnia disappeared. I no longer have to wear socks to bed; I feel comfortably warm. My son's chronic heartburn and eczema disappeared."*

A.B. says *"IBS is pretty much gone. Eczema, too. And mood swings, mostly."*

L.P. says *"Don't have to eat all the time or dream about chocolate. No stomach pains or feeling like death after eating too much. Stronger fingernails and hair, more energy and better sleep."*

A.W. says *"No more chronic heartburn.... and apparently I'm allergic to carbs, or wheat or something...I used to get itching at night... not any more..."*

A.T.W. says *"food no longer has any control over my life...."*

C.C. says *"Chronic pain almost nonexistent. Skin got better. Sleeping better, mood regulation better."*

P.B. says *"My sleep is still crazy messed up, but i eat a lot less. I used to be too nauseous in the mornings to eat, but then light headed and* sick in the afternoon cause I hadn't eaten. Blood pressure is down, few other things."

C.D. says *"It controls the symptoms of my auto immune disease to the point that my chronic pain is gone. I hardly ever feel hungry and don't get cravings. I have more energy."*

P.T. says *"My auto immune related joint pain is about 90% better, my psoriasis, which I've had consistently since I was a teenager, is about 50% gone, my moods have never been more stable and I'm sleeping normally for the first time in seven years. The weight loss has become least important to me on the list of benefits!"*

C.D. also replies that *"I have RA and a non specified auto immune disease, lupus like illness with costochondritis. The diet really reduces my inflammation."*

W.D. says *"No more IBS, migraines, or hangovers for me."*

M.L. says *"Off thyroid meds and endless amounts of energy. I used to collapse at 9 pm get cranky and sleep minimum of 8 hours. Now I'm rarely ever tired but almost still have trouble sleeping. And the body composition changes are amazing."*

C.B.P. says *"I felt clear headed and though I didn't lose much weight, I lost inches. Also, really soft skin."*

E.S. (talking about her child) says *"No seizures. That's it and we have to watch calories or C gets fat and given we have to lift her as she has cerebral palsy this is not a good thing. She had hundreds and severe cognitive regression. Now she has been seizure free on the keto for 5 years and is 'normal' cognitively."*

I.K. says *"After 15 days my blood sugar measures show normal results, I could cut my insulin input by two thirds. I feel great and of course lost more than 9 pounds right now!"*

These are only a few of the comments that I'm showing you from my small unorganized Facebook poll. So, most of these people report:

reduced inflammation, higher energy levels, better sleep, reduced seizures, better control over blood sugar levels, and reduced cravings.

In the following chapter I'm going to talk about insulin resistance, diabetes, obesity, and the metabolic syndrome. I'm also going to talk about the use of ketogenic diets for medical conditions such as the treatment of epilepsy, reduction of inflammation, and the emergence of studies relating to the treatment of cancer.

Chapter Five

Health Implications of Ketogenic Nutrition

Insulin Resistance, Diabetes, and Obesity

Remember that I've told you about our ancestors who did not have access to foods with such high concentrations of carbohydrates. Grains only came around ~10,000 years ago. This is the Paleolithic argument for high fat nutrition.

10,000 years in the context of human evolution of more than 2 million years is a mere glimpse. Throughout this entire period of 2 million years, we were mostly consuming high fat nutrition. Yes, we did consume some fruits and vegetables, but they were not available in all seasons. Besides, the context was different. People were not sedentary like they are today.

I cannot imagine that our fellow Paleolithic counterparts stayed all day in the cave watching Paleo TV. Nor can I picture them behind their desks doing Paleo paperwork for more than 8 hours straight. They were likely moving all day searching for food. You see, the context is very different.

Paradoxically the worst and the best period of human evolution is the past 100 years. We've seen the technological boom, we've become more civilized, we've cured a lot of diseases, but we've also gained other diseases.

We've increased our life span, yet what's the purpose of this longer life-span if we cannot live it in a very enjoyable fashion? What's the purpose of living 70 years if once you pass the 50+ mark you start taking medications for all sorts of health issues?

We're not yet genetically adapted to process the big amounts of carbohydrates we consume. Adding fat in the context of high carb is even worse. Phinney [5] says that a high fat diet starts somewhere at 60% of the calories coming from fat and less than 10% of them coming from carbohydrates. Yet, we've seen a lot of research studies demonizing fat intake by comparing high-carb diets with high-fat diets. And these high-fat diets were 30-50% fat, 20-30% carbs, and the rest of the calories were protein.

Sadly, we are imparting the same life habits to our children. They do not spend too much time outside and when they do they have their gadgets at hand. Stop for a second and think about it. Next time you're outdoors, take a moment and look around you. How many people have their smartphones in their hands? While you're at the coffee shop, how many people are frenetically tickling the glass of their mobile devices? I would not even consider EM radiation because if you put that into context (which I believe is very important), things are even worse.

This continuous connectivity makes us even more sedentary. Don't get me wrong here. The other side of the equation is not good either. If you spend 2 hours in the gym everyday exhausting yourself, you're basically pushing the self-destruct button. Exercising should be done for the health of the mind, for improved concentration, and for general well being, not for weight loss.

Doug McGuff's book *Body by Science* [30] clearly describes efficient exercise using hundreds of research articles and his 25+ years of experience in the field of exercise physiology. I've started applying his teachings which are based on the premise: "workout less - gain more" and so far it's been working great for me. I'll talk more about his protocols and *The Big Five* training regimen in the chapter dedicated to very low-carb performance.

The increased intake of refined carbohydrates contributed to the epidemics of obesity and diabetes. The metabolic syndrome made its appearance in the past 50 years and it is characterized by: central obesity, increased levels of fasting blood glucose, high-blood pressure, increased levels of triglycerides in the blood as well as low HDL cholesterol. This metabolic syndrome increases the risk of heart failure as well as diabetes and obesity.

Proponents of high-fat nutrition propose that insulin resistance leads to this problem. Now, let's try to understand this concept.

Insulin resistance basically occurs when the insulin released from the pancreas cannot handle the amount of glucose in the blood. This is because the insulin receptors from your cells do not respond to insulin's action efficiently.

Under normal conditions insulin attaches to the insulin receptors of the cells inside the body, which allows the entrance of glucose inside the cell for energy production. But when you are insulin resistant, your pancreas needs to over-shoot insulin for the same levels of glucose because the insulin receptors from the cell are less activated by insulin. Thus, glucose will not enter the cell efficiently.

In this context, the levels of glucose within the blood are elevated and this triggers the secretion of even more insulin to try to reduce blood glucose levels. It is a vicious circle [31]. Let me try to explain it as simply as I can:

Insulin resistance occurs when "normal or elevated insulin levels" cannot efficiently dispose glucose from the blood.

Why does this happen? Because your cells have lost their capacity to react to insulin.

In type 2 diabetes the human body is insulin resistant which means it does not properly use the insulin it produces. The high blood sugar signalizes the pancreas to secrete more insulin but this process cannot continue indefinitely because the pancreas cannot keep up with the rising demands for insulin. Patients suffering from T2D are advised to change their diets and are encouraged to exercise, and they ultimately take metformin (to increase insulin sensitivity) or, eventually, even insulin.

Conversely, in type 1 diabetes, the human body cannot produce insulin because there is an autoimmune response which attacks the beta-cells in the pancreas. These beta-cells are the ones that produce insulin. Patients suffering from T1D have to be administered insulin to keep the blood sugar levels normal.

Sadly, ADA [33] promotes the use of fruits, whole grains, and low fat foods in the management of diabetes. These types of foods cause an insulin response the same way that high carbohydrate foods cause. For example 1 medium size apple is 11g of carbohydrates. Eat that and 2-3 slices of whole grain bread in the morning and your insulin levels will go up.

I'm not sure why it takes so long for ADA to admit that carbohydrates have to strictly be limited in diabetes, while nutrition needs to be focused around fatty foods, especially healthy fats (avoid vegetable oils). According to ADA (2014) [33], a diabetic patient should target 45-60 grams of carbohydrate per meal. Eat three meals per day and you'll have 150-180 grams of carbohydrate intake. That's insane. Ketogenic diets target 30 grams of net carbohydrates per day.

Since the diabetic is not able to efficiently use insulin to lower blood glucose, the body will respond by increasing insulin production. Since glucose cannot efficiently enter into the cells, the body is deprived of energy. Hunger is present most of the time. The body tries to excrete glucose through urine. It needs a lot of water to do so, which is why the diabetic will feel thirst.

The situation is even worse in T1D (type 1 diabetes) because the patient would need a lot of exogenous (outside of the body) insulin to be injected to be able to maintain normal blood glucose levels in the context of 150-180g of carbohydrate intake per day.

How can we stop the cascade of these negative effects from happening? By lowering blood glucose levels.

And how do you do that? By lowering the intake of carbohydrates.

If you eat very few carbohydrates, where do you get your energy from? You have to increase the intake of fat and allow your body to adapt to using fat as a primary source of energy.

As you start lowering blood glucose levels by reducing the intake of carbohydrates, there will be less secretion of insulin. If you do this on a consistent basis, your cells may recover their sensitivity to insulin. Even if this happens, why should you start increasing the ingestion of carbohydrates? (aka: why not making this a way of living? and not a diet).

If you lower the intake of carbs (<50g/day) and increase the intake of fat and if you do it for a certain period of time, your body will adapt to using fat as a primary source of fuel and will not require glucose as it is required in a glucose dependent metabolism. Insulin secretion will be lowered.

If you eat more than your body needs for energy, your body stores the excess of nutrients that you ingested. For example if you eat 2500 kcals in a day and your body only uses 2000 kcals, the rest of them will be stored as body fat. I am talking in the context of a carbohydrate rich diet.

So, if most of the calories you ingest come from carbohydrates, the excess of carbohydrates that are not needed will be turned into fat through the process of lipogenesis. Let's look at it from a different perspective.

Glucose uptake by the cells is stimulated by insulin. When the cells have all the glucose they need, insulin promotes lipogenesis (conversion of carbohydrates to fats and mobilization of these fats into adipocytes) [31] and it suppresses lipolysis (release of fat from the adipose tissue).

Lipolysis usually occurs when the body runs of out glucose for the production of energy. It happens by mobilizing fat from adipocytes and converting them to ketone bodies (which are then used for energy production) [32].

Nowadays, it becomes easier to eat more than the body needs. While many of us are sedentary, our basal metabolic rates are lower. This means that we need less energy (as total calories) to make it through the day. We have rich carbohydrate sources at hand everywhere.

The supermarkets are loaded with sugary foods. There are sugars even in the foods that we would not suspect them to be in. There is sugar in meats; there is a lot of sugar in the dairy products. And the saddest of all is that there is a lot sugar (carbohydrates) in diabetics' products.

Here's a simple comparison on two similar products, one being labeled as "sugar free".

CHOCOLATE CHIP COOKIES

Nutrition Facts	Amount/serving	%DV*	Amount/serving	%DV*
Serv. Size 1 cookie (25g)	**Total Fat** 4.5g	7%	**Total Carb.** 16g	5%
Servings 8	Sat. Fat 1.5g	9%	Fiber 1g	2%
Calories 110 Fat Cal. 40	*Trans* Fat 0g		Sugars 9g	
	Cholest. 0mg	0%	**Protein** 1g	
*Percent Daily Values (DV) are based on a 2,000 calorie diet.	**Sodium** 60mg	2%		
	Vitamin A 0% • Vitamin C 0% • Calcium 0% • Iron 4%			

Ingredients: Spelt (Wheat)* Flour, Non-Hydrogenated Expeller-Pressed Oils (Soybean, Palm Fruit, Canola, Olive, Soy Protein (Soy), Soy Lecithin, Natural Flavor From Corn, Non-Dairy Lactic Acid From Beets, Natural Beta-Carotene Color), Evaporated Cane Juice, Brown Sugar, Semi-Sweet Chocolate Chips (Sugar, Chocolate Liquor, Non-Dairy Cocoa Butter, Dextrose, Soy Lecithin, Vanilla) Vanilla Flavor (Dextrose, Natural Flavors), Vegan Butterscotch Flavor (Dextrose, Natural Flavors), Baking Soda, Xanthan Gum.

and the "sugar free" one:

Sugar Free Cookies
Chocolate

Nutrition Facts	Amount Per Serving	%DV*	Amount Per Serving	%DV*
Serving Size 3 Cookies (28g)	**Total Fat** 7g	11%	**Total Carbohydrate** 19g	6%
Servings Per Container About 6	Saturated Fat 2.5g	13%	Dietary Fiber 1g	4%
	Trans Fat 0g		Sugars 0g	
Calories 130	**Cholesterol** 0mg	0%	Sugar Alcohol 6g	
Calories from Fat 60	**Sodium** 55mg	2%	**Protein** 1g	
*Percent Daily Values (DV) are based on a 2,000 calorie diet.	Vitamin A 0% • Vitamin C 0% • Calcium 0% • Iron 6%			

INGREDIENTS: ENRICHED FLOUR (WHEAT FLOUR, NIACIN, REDUCED IRON, THIAMIN MONONITRATE [VITAMIN B₁], RIBOFLAVIN [VITAMIN B₂], FOLIC ACID), VEGETABLE OIL (SOYBEAN, PALM AND PALM KERNEL OIL WITH TBHQ FOR FRESHNESS), SORBITOL*, MALTODEXTRIN, COCOA (PROCESSED WITH ALKALI), POLYDEXTROSE, CORNSTARCH, LACTITOL, CONTAINS TWO PERCENT OR LESS OF NATURAL AND ARTIFICIAL FLAVOR, WHEY PROTEIN CONCENTRATE, SALT, LEAVENING (BAKING SODA, MONOCALCIUM PHOSPHATE), SOY LECITHIN, CHOCOLATE, ACESULFAME POTASSIUM, COLOR ADDED, DATEM, SUCRALOSE, ANNATTO COLOR.
*EXCESS CONSUMPTION MAY HAVE A LAXATIVE EFFECT.   CONTAINS WHEAT, MILK AND SOY INGREDIENTS, MAY CONTAIN TRACES OF PEANUT.

Now let's examine the facts:

The total carbohydrate count per 100 grams (fair serving) for the first one is 64 grams, while for the second one (the "sugar free") is 68 grams.

What the heck? The "sugar free" one contains more total carbohydrates than the regular one. The amount of fiber is approximately the same in both of them.

Even though the sugar free one does not contain table sugar it contains a lot of different ingredients which produce spikes in the insulin levels.

What would enriched flour, cornstarch, and polydextrose have to do with "sugar free products"?

Please be careful at what you're buying if you're diabetic. Make sure that the net carbohydrate count is very low (net carbs = total carbs - fiber) and make sure it fits into your < 30g of net carbohydrates per day. Here's a good example of dark chocolate 85% cocoa:

Nährwerte / Nutritional value	Ø pro/ per 100 g/	Ø pro/ per Riegel/ per serving (20 g)	% GDA*
Brennwert/ Energy	2468 kJ / 598 kcal	494 kJ / 120 kcal	6 %
Eiweiss/ Protein	8,2 g	1,6 g	3 %
Kohlenhydrate/Carbohydrate	14,7 g	2,9 g	1 %
davon Zucker/ of which sugar	14,0 g	2,8 g	3 %
Fett/ Fat	53,3 g	10,7 g	15 %
davon gesättigte Fettsäuren/ of which saturates	33,6 g	6,7 g	34 %
Ballaststoffe/ Fibres	13,1 g	2,6 g	11 %
Natrium/ Sodium	0,01 g	0,00 g	0 %
*der empf. Tagesmenge / of an adult's guideline daily amount.			

You can see that the net carbohydrate is 14.7g per 100g in this case. They did not include the fibers in the carbohydrate count here. The fibers are listed as well, so the "Carbohydrate" is actually the "net carbohydrates". Conversely, normal chocolate as well as many "diabetic" chocolates have 50-60 grams of net carbohydrates per 100g in their carb count.

You could eat an entire 100g chocolate like the one above as it would only have ~15g of net carbohydrates if the rest of the net carbs you consume do not exceed the 30g/day mark. The ingredients of this chocolate say: cocoa butter, cocoa mass, and sugar. Even though it has sugar in it, the amount of sugar is very low and does not have an impact on insulin levels in this context.

The good news is that very low carbohydrate diets have consistently proved and keep proving that diabetes can be well managed and even reversed as the work of Phinney and Volek [5] shows.

Here's what CDC [39] reported in 2011 with respect to diabetes rates over a period of 30 years:

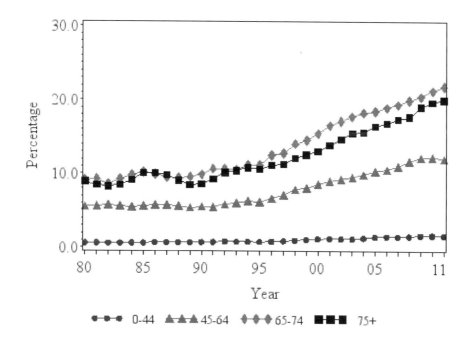

Let's analyze the facts. You can see there is only a slight increase in incidence rates for the population of age 0 to 44. However, things are dramatic when you look at the population age above 44 years. There are a lot of reasons that would explain it. I would mostly attribute this higher incidence of diabetes to the slower metabolic rate, to a more sedentary life (people are not as active as they were when they were younger), as well as to food intake habits (which is probably the most controllable and most important aspect).

There is another CDC report [40] from 2012 which follows historic data of diabetes, specifically: Annual Number of New Cases of Diagnosed Diabetes Among U.S. Adults Aged 18-79 years, from 1980 to 2010. Here's the statistic:

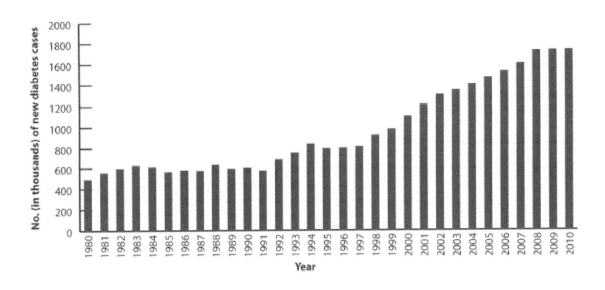

We should think of these numbers in the context of the dietary guidelines which have been pushed down our throat for the past 40 years. I'm not sure if you know, but we've been promoting a high-carb nutritional plan (6+ servings of grain products + 4+ servings of fruits and vegetables at the base of the pyramid) ever since the 1970s. Call that healthy eating!

If we continue on the current path, here's what the Assistant Secretary for Planning and Evaluation from the U.S. Department of Health and Human Service is predicting [41]:

Diagnosed (1960-1998) and Projected Diagnosed (2000-2050) Cases

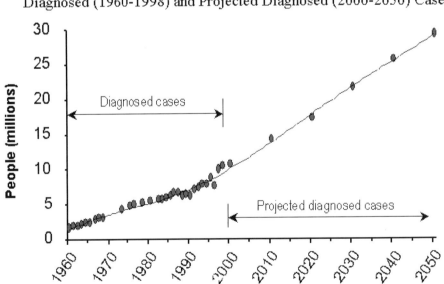

The entire population is growing obese. I don't want to be panicky but do you really think that this whole fear of fat and this entire elimination of fat (at least in the dietary guidelines) from our nutrition while increasing the amount of carbohydrates is doing us any good?

Current predictions are for an increase from 11 million in 2000 to 29 million people diagnosed with diabetes by 2050. This is an increase of 165%. The complications that are associated with diabetes are: blindness, kidney failure, amputations, and cardiovascular disease deaths [41].

The person reading this tends to look at the statistic thinking that they have nothing to do with it. But, why would you be excluded from this statistic?

Are you doing something different? Are you not eating the usual bagel at 10 A.M. in the office? Are you not having the healthy cereal and milk breakfast? Or toast with orange juice?

One thing that is important to know is that Type 2 Diabetes does not occur over night. It is a slow steady process that lasts for several years and it often is diagnosed 6-7 years after being triggered. There are a lot of signs that tell you whether or not you've started developing insulin resistance. However, the best thing to do would be to keep insulin levels as low as possible and you do this by drastically decreasing the amount of carbohydrates you ingest (by now, you know that very well). We've seen the big picture of diabetes. Now, let's dig deeper into some research studies.

In this study [34] done by Westman and colleagues in 2007, the researchers conducted a review on the health implications of very low carbohydrate (ketogenic) diets. They mentioned a study of 10 subjects that were obese and had T2D (type 2 diabetes). They were monitored while eating their usual diet for 7 days and then a very low carbohydrate diet for 14 days. Their carbohydrate intake was lowered to 21 grams per day. However, the subjects were allowed to eat as much protein and fat as they wanted.

They consumed an average of: 164 grams of fat, 21g of carbohydrates and 151 grams of protein. This translates to ~2164 kcals per day. Their normal diet (observed in the 7d period) consisted of ~3100kcals. This means that the subjects lowered their energy intake by more than 900kcals. They lost ~2kg over a period of 14 days. The mean fasting glucose was decreased from 135mg/dL to 113mg/dL, Hba1c (glycated hemoglobin) was decreased from 7.3% to 6.8%, while blood glucose and insulin concentrations significantly decreased. 5 out of the 10 patients reduced their diabetes medication as a result.

Another study [35] followed 40 subjects with atherogenic dyslipidemia (a disorder in the metabolism of lipoproteins) for 12 weeks. They were divided into two groups. Both of the groups were put on hypocaloric diets of 1500 kcals/day.

The first group was the CRD group (carbohydrate restricted diet) in which the percentage of calories was broken down as follows:

12% - carbohydrate
59% - fat
28% - protein

The second group was the LFD group (low fat diet) in which the percentage of calories was broken down as follows:

56% - carbohydrate
24% - fat
20% - protein

The researchers observed that various metabolic markers improved in both groups, but the CRD group had more consistent results: -12% blood glucose, -50% insulin levels, 55% better insulin sensitivity, -10% more weight loss, -14% adiposity, -51% TAG (triacylglycerol), +13% HDL-C (good cholesterol), and other improvements. Note that the CRD group's saturated fat intake was three times bigger than the other group. The researchers concluded that restricting carbohydrates is a very efficient way to improve the features of the Metabolic Syndrome as well as to reduce the risk of cardiovascular disease.

In another study [36] Westman and colleagues wanted to determine the impact of a low-carbohydrate (ketogenic) diet vs. a low-glycemic index diet on T2D. The research followed 84 volunteers with T2D and obesity who were randomized into two groups: the ketogenic diet group LCKD, and a low-glycemic-low-calorie group LGID. The main purpose of the study was to control blood glucose levels and this was measured by HbA1c (glycated hemoglobin).

HbA1c measures the average blood glucose concentration over a certain period of time. It shows the level of attachment of glucose on hemoglobin over a maximum of three to four months, which is the lifespan of hemoglobin.

In this study [36] both groups showed improvements in bio-markers, such as: HbA1c, fasting insulin levels, fasting blood glucose levels, as well as in weight loss. However, the LCKD group had shown better improvements compared to the other group:

HbA1c -1.5% in LCKD compared to -0.5% in LGID
Weight -11.1kg in LCKD compared to -6.9kg in LGID
HDL-C +5.6mg/dL in LCKD compared to no change in LGID
Diabetes medications -95.2% in LCKD compared to -62% in LGID

In another study [37] Yancy and colleagues recruited 28 overweight participants who had T2D. The experiment lasted for 16 weeks and they were put on a <20g carb/day diet. 21 of the 28 patients have completed the study and I think this shows a very good compliance with the experiment compared to other approaches that use low-calorie high-carbohydrate diets.

The researchers have measured HbA1c and observed that it decreased by 16% at the end of the experiment (from ~7.5% to 6.3%). 7 patients have stopped using their diabetes medications, 10 patients have reduced their dosage, while 4 patients have kept the dose unchanged. The average bodyweight decrease was 6.6% (from 131kg to 123kg). Fasting serum triglycerides decreased by 42%, while other lipid measurements did not change significantly.

In another study [38] Dashti and colleagues followed 64 obese but healthy individuals (BMI > 30), out of which some of them (31 subjects) had high blood glucose levels. The subjects were put on a ketogenic diet and were followed for 56 weeks. The researchers took various measures at weeks 0, 8, 16, 24, 48, and 56. They measured: BMI, body weight, blood glucose levels, total cholesterol, LDL-cholesterol, HDL-cholesterol, triglycerides, urea, and creatinine.

According to the researchers [38], the body weight, BMI, glucose levels, total cholesterol, LDL-c, TAG, and urea showed a significant decrease from week 1 to week 56, whereas the levels of HDL-c increased significantly. They also noticed that the changes were more significant for the group with high blood glucose levels. Creatinine level changes have not been significant.

In this case the researchers concluded that ketogenic diets have beneficial effects in obese diabetic subjects as long as they are followed over the long-term. The long-term use of the ketogenic diet is safe, as per the researchers' conclusions. Now let's talk about fat accumulation.

Insulin, Obesity and LPL

T2D and obesity often come into a single package. They are closely correlated. High blood glucose levels promote fat accumulation into adipocytes because insulin is not able to get glucose into the cells for energy production, since the cells have become insulin resistant.

Thus, the excess glucose has nowhere to go but to being packed into triglycerides and stored as fat through the process of lipogenesis. The fact that glucose cannot get inside the cell triggers the pancreas to secrete more insulin. Some of the glucose is excreted through urine, but still, the blood sugar levels remain high enough.

It is hard to understand the reasoning for insulin administration as well as drug intake in T2D. Why would you want to eliminate the effect of something (high glucose levels) and do it for indefinite periods of time when you should focus on ameliorating the cause (reducing carbohydrate intake)?

Why would folks want to over-exercise if they are obese, but make no changes to their eating patterns?

They would not achieve anything, except sore muscles!

Enter LPL and Leptin

The entire obesity equation and the fat accumulation process is much more than the calories-in versus calories-out theorem. There are many hormones that impact the general state of well being of the human body (homeostasis). Gary Taubes explains it very well in his book *Good Calories Bad Calories* [16].

LPL is the short form of lipoprotein lipase. This is an enzyme (of which many people have not heard of) that is found both on adipocytes and on muscle cells. When LPL is activated on the surface of the fat cell, it will promote fat accumulation. Conversely, when LPL is activated on the surface of muscle cell it will promote fat uptake by the muscle cell for the purpose of oxidation to generate energy.

Peter Attia [2] thinks that as humans age, they tend to have less LPL on muscle cells and more LPL on fat cells. Both of these processes are promoters of fat accumulation.

It has been theorized that the activity of LPL is modulated partially by the levels of insulin within the plasma. In this study [42] from 2012 the researchers wanted to find out the effects that hyperinsulinemia has on LPL activity on muscle, adipose tissue, and on postheparin plasma.

Subjects were divided into three groups: young-healthy (YS), older with T2D (DS), and older control subjects (CS). Researchers noted that the effect of insulin on LPL leads to an increase of 20 to 30% activity in the adipose tissues and a decrease of 20 to 25% in postheparin plasma. Remember that higher LPL activity on fat cells promotes fat accumulation.

Various studies [43] have also suggested that LPL activity in adipose tissue is stimulated by insulin and that higher plasma insulin levels decrease the activity of LPL on muscle tissue.

In fact, an older study conducted in 1982 [44] followed subjects who were put on carbohydrate rich diets where 80% of the energy was taken from carbs. The researchers observed that higher plasma insulin levels was associated with a significant (-55%) decrease in the activity of LPL on muscle cells compared to a control group.

The key take-away on lipoprotein lipase (LPL) is according to Peter Attia [45] that insulin up-regulates (increases the activity of) LPL on adipocytes (fat-cells) and down-regulates (decreases the activity of) LPL on lean tissue (muscle-cells).

It means that when insulin levels are high, more LPL will be activated on fat-cells promoting fat accumulation and less LPL will be activated on muscle cells, preventing fat oxidation by the muscle. So, it would seem advantageous to maintain lower insulin levels.

Another important hormone in the context of fat accumulation and obesity is leptin. According to Kulik-Rechberger [46], this is a hormone mainly released by adipocytes. So it is made in our fat cells. One of its functions is to regulate energy balance by lowering food intake and increasing energy expenditure. So, its target is homeostasis (general well being).

This should be very simply understood. Leptin secretion is directly proportional with fat tissue. Thus, the more fat tissue, the more leptin secretion.

What does leptin secretion mean?

It basically means that when your fat cells release leptin into the body they go into your brain (hypothalamus) via the bloodstream. They signal that there's enough fat in the body (i.e. now it's time to stop eating). The thyroid gland is involved into this process as well.

This is a very complicated equation and it is even so in overweight individuals because their high leptin levels cannot efficiently signal the hypothalamus to lower the appetite so the body keeps accumulating fat. So as you become fatter, you'll tend to eat more and become even fatter.

This is when your body becomes leptin resistant. Insulin resistance and leptin resistance are tied together and according to Dr. Jack Kruse

[47] leptin resistance occurs 5-7 years before insulin resistance occurs. So, you'd be able to tell whether or not you are likely to develop T2D if you are leptin resistant. Dr. Kruse is of the opinion that high-leptin levels destroy a protein (amylin) in the beta cells of the pancreas. Thus, the beta cells will become inefficient at producing insulin. Correlate that with higher blood glucose as a result of a high-carbohydrate diet and you have the perfect recipe for T2D.

The work and research of Dr. Jack Kruse [47] on leptin is amazing. There's no point for me to go into further details on this topic because Dr. Kruse covers it extremely well in his book [48] and on his website. However, the key take-away on how to increase leptin sensitivity is, as you may have guessed, drastically decrease the intake of carbohydrates. This should restore your normal leptin efficiency in a matter of weeks. You could also apply the CT protocol of Jack Kruse and do some HIIT Training, but I'll tell you more about that later.

Saturated Fat - Is this the real culprit?

Proponents of ketogenic diets have long known that there is no correlation between saturated fat intake and health issues like cardiovascular disease. However, once the evil has been released, it is difficult to try and fix things. Once people have started to believe that saturated fat will cause heart issues, it is not easy to change their minds. This message is still promoted by the media throughout the world. People are advised to avoid all fats in their diets.

The United States' dietary guidelines have been promoting a very low fat diet for more than 30 years now. And what do we see as a result of that?

An ever increasing waist size and higher obesity rates as the years pass. The origin of this was the erroneous and misleading interpretations of Ancel Keys in his studies.

Ancel Keys was a scientist of the 20th century who studied the effect of nutrition on health (among others). He focused mostly on how dietary fat intake impacts prevalence of cardio-vascular disease. He conducted research on 22 countries where he showed the correlation between intake of fat and heart disease. However, he did not present all the 22 countries that he studied. He only showed 7 countries that fit in his research.

It was later found out that Keys' conclusions on the research were not valid when all 22 countries were considered. In fact it showed that there was no correlation between intake of fat and cardio-vascular disease. Here's the initial data published by Keys himself [50]:

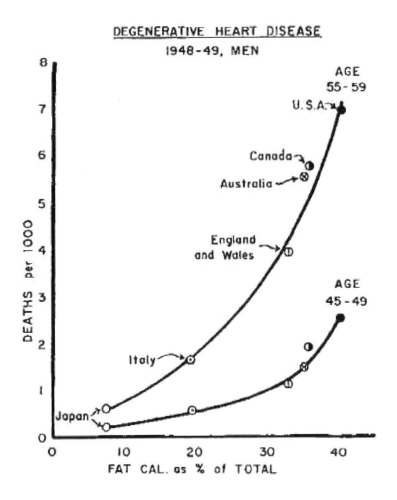

If you look at the graph you can conclude that the higher the fat intake, the larger the number of deaths from heart disease. Keys was a very influential man and his studies contributed to the enactment of the general dietary guidelines in the United States. The first issue of them was entitled: Dietary Goals for the United States [51] and they promoted a consumption of 55-60% of calories as carbohydrates from the total daily caloric intake along with drastic reduction in fat intake.

Keys started preaching about his findings in 1955 and as you can see in the diagram the data was from 1948-1949. However, two years later in 1957, two researchers re-analyzed Keys' research and published their findings showing all the 22 countries that Keys did not include in his study [52]. Here's what the "real" data looked like:

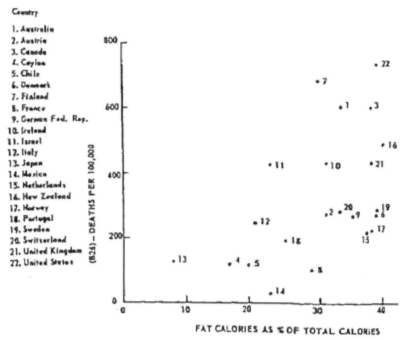

FIG. 3. Mortality from arteriosclerotic and degenerative heart disease (B-26) and fat calories as per cent of total calories in males fifty-five to fifty-nine years. Calculated from national food balance data by F.A.O. (see text for definition).

Yerushalmy and Hilleboe [52] were granted access to the same databases that Ancel Keys had and their diagram tells a different story. If you see the data from a bigger perspective you can see that there's no correlation between fat intake and cardio-vascular disease. Even if we know that and even if it was known ever since Yerushalmy and Hilleboe have pointed it out in 1957, the general guidelines still promote a very low fat intake and a high-carbohydrate intake.

Would you find that as a rational thing to do?

If you think in terms of big industries and politics, yes.

Throughout these past few decades there have been countless of studies proving the contrary: no direct correlation between fat intake and cardio-vascular problems. There is this meta-analysis [53] from 2010.

Meta-analyses are observational studies that analyze various research studies conducted with the same or similar purposes to test a certain hypothesis. They're basically studies of studies.

The objective of the meta-analysis [53] from 2010 was to provide a summary of the evidence related to the association of fat intake and CHD (coronary heart disease), stroke, as well as CVD (cardio-vascular disease).

There were 21 studies in this meta-analysis which followed ~348,000 subjects over periods of 5 to 23 years. The meta-analysis reached the conclusion that there is no significant proof to associate the intake of saturated fat with a higher risk of CVD and/or CHD.

Even though it is not easy to conduct good research studies because there are too many variables to analyze, Ancel Keys would have done much of a better job if he would have considered at least the carbohydrate intake as an important factor in his studies.

Here's for example a very recent study [55] showing why people still fall for the "fat is bad" myth. It was released in February 2014 and it followed 39 young normal weight individuals who overfed on saturated or polyunsaturated fat. The groups overfeeding with saturated fat consumed muffins high in palm oil (Saturated Fat - SFA) or sunflower oil (Polyunsaturated Fat - PUFA) for a period of 7 weeks.

Do I have to proceed further with the explanation? Really? Muffins?

And they called it a high-fat diet [55]. So, the researchers assessed visceral fat, liver fat, total adipose tissue, as well as subcutaneous abdominal fat, pancreatic fat, and lean tissue. They observed that both of the groups gained similar weight but that the SFA group has shown higher liver fat and visceral fat while the PUFA group has shown higher lean tissue after overfeeding. They concluded that SFA over-consumption leads to visceral fat storage while PUFA promotes lean tissue accumulation.

I see this as a very poorly conducted research study because they never mention anything about carbohydrate consumption in both of the groups (muffins are high-carb). The sad part is that I've seen smart individuals from the keto community who fell for it. I also fell for it in the beginning but then I re-read it a few times until I saw the magic word "muffins". I was desperately over the confirmation bias again :).

Aaaa, what a delight! You can never over-eat muffins, they're so rich in both carbs and fats that consuming them will spike your insulin levels and you'll keep desiring more. This is bad science or this is only my biased thinking. Either one is good for me.

Phinney and Volek [5] always say that fat intake is bad for health when the % of calories from fat is < 60% and the carbohydrate intake is high.

For example, a diet made of 40% fat, 40% carbohydrates, and 20% protein can cause a lot of health issues. Many research studies consider high-fat-low-carb diets as being: 40%-60% fat, 20-30% carbs, 20-30% protein. That is why they should not be considered relevant.

A good high-fat diet is one that is high in fat (more than 60% from total calories) and very low in carbohydrates (less than 10%). Make sure you know this when analyzing research studies.

When there is a higher % of both fat and carbohydrates in the diet, your body will choose to use glucose as primary fuel, while all the fat will get into the adipose tissue. Besides, the excess carbohydrates will also go into the fat tissue through lipogenesis (conversion of carbohydrates into fats). High-insulin levels promote fat accumulation and since there is a high-carbohydrate intake, the constant hunger will promote the ingestion of more food of the same kind and less oxidation of fat [54].

Think of it like going to a fast-food restaurant and having a big-burger with fries and soda. The burger and fries are high-fat-high-carb, while the soda is high-carb. No wonder you are hungry 3-4 hours after this kind of meal, given that you ingested 1000+ kcals.

In the same context of 1000+ kcals per day (not per meal) a keto-adapted person can lose weight without ever feeling hungry. This is why macro partitioning really matters.

Let's see the historical obesity prevalence ever since the low fat dogma has been thrown down our esophagus. Thanks Dr. Mercola for the diagram below.

Prevalence of Obesity Among U.S. Adults Aged 20-74

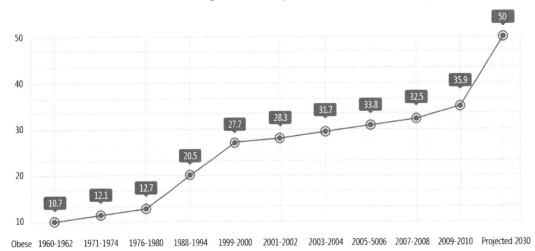

Derived from NHANES data (http://www.cdc.gov/nchs/data/hestat/obesity_adult_09_10/obesity_adult_09_10.html#table1)

Remember that Ancel Keys was a very influential man and that the dietary guidelines back from the 70s have a lot to do with his amazing research that demonized fat intake. Those dietary guidelines promoted higher carbohydrate intake and less consumption of fat.

The same USDA dietary guidelines have been reconsidered several times ever since, and in the 1980s they promoted the drastic reduction of all types of fats [56] and the need for a higher consumption of complex carbohydrates and fiber. According to Pennington and Baker [57], other than contribution to dental caries there is no significant evidence that sugars demonstrate a hazard to general public "when sugars are consumed at the levels" that are now current and in the manner now practiced.

I guess these guys were really delusional. The data in the graph above was available in the 1990s as well, and those were the times that obesity and diabetes were at high peaks. I try to find the logic behind their reasoning. My thinking may be biased but let me try to think in terms of the bad science that I referred to above.

I know that it's not all about carbohydrate intake. There are other important variables in the complex equation of general health. But carbohydrate intake has a significant contribution, if you ask me.

I am really into the ketogenic lifestyle because I found tremendous health benefits other than just fat loss, compared to the time when I was following a moderate to high carbohydrate diet with lower fat intake. Now, that I found my holy grail of nutrition, I'm promoting high-fat nutrition. So, I may think in terms of this single variable: increased fat intake. But, again, I know that it's more than that: you have to go very low on carbohydrate to reap the benefits.

And you will start seeing these benefits after an adaptation period of a couple of weeks. Few people are willing to go for it. The sports community demolishes this dogma from the ground up. I may be biased but I want to think in terms of high-fat very low carbohydrate. It works extremely well for me and I know it works for many people who have the courage necessary to say no to others pushing carbohydrates all over the place: at work, in the supermarket, at home, etc.

This is one of the reasons that many people do not succeed on very low-carb-high-fat ketogenic diets. They are not strong enough to fight back public influence. I don't want to get away from the subject, so I'm asking the same question again.

If the keto community considers a high-fat diet as being one with 60%+ fat and less than 10% carbs, why do scientists and researchers do not take this prescription when labeling their experiments as "high-fat" vs. (whatever you want to fill it in here).? Why?

Why there is so little research conducted using this type of high-fat prescription? I know there is a big battle to be taken.

I'm going "all-in" because I cannot stand seeing diabetes and obesity ever increasing. I cannot stand seeing people suffering from all types of illnesses and disorders which derive from inflammation. I cannot stand seeing overweight people going on the treadmill and exhausting themselves without seeing any results...And I cannot stand seeing them give up.

This has to stop. I don't want the predictions from above to become true.

A better story of Saturated Fatty Acids

My thinking is based on Phinney's [5] experiments on the correlation between saturated fat and low carbohydrate intake. Let's see another side of the coin.

Phinney and 12 other researchers [58] have shown that a hypocaloric carbohydrate restricted diet (very-low-carb-low-calorie diet) has two major health benefits, such as reduced levels of saturated fatty acids in the blood (even though the intake of saturated fatty acids is increased) compared to a low fat diet and it reduced inflammation even though arachidonic acid was increased.

They gave 8 healthy subjects CRD (carbohydrate-restricted diets) for 6 weeks. There were two diets, one that was higher in saturated fat and the other that was higher in unsaturated fat. Both of the groups have shown lower TAG (triglycerides), lower insulin levels, and higher LDL-C (yes, LDL-C the "bad" one). Both of the groups have shown lower POA which is palmitoleic acid. This type of acid is indicative of lipogenesis and it could be a very good indicator of diabetes and obesity, way before insulin resistance takes place. The researchers point out that saturated fat is properly metabolized when carbohydrate is restricted.

Phinney and Volek [5] always draw attention to the fact that saturated fat intake may not matter in the context of a well formulated low-carbohydrate diet because they have shown that saturated fatty acids are preferably burned in beta-oxidation over poly-unsaturated fatty acids and mono-unsaturated fatty acids. This means that if you eat saturated fat on a ketogenic diet, you will preferably burn that saturated fat first.

The major drawback with these types of research studies when ketogenic subjects are followed is that is not easy to recruit people into them. Once on a ketogenic diet, it is easy to sustain it. Take for example the A to Z study from 2008 in which Christopher Gardner [59] compared 4 diets (Atkins, Learn, Ornish, and Zone) for a 1 year period. A number of 311 subjects have been divided into the 4 groups, each group following a particular diet.

In this case the group with the biggest retention of subjects throughout the entire period of a year was the Atkins group, with 88% of the subjects sticking through the end (compliance), followed up by the Ornish group with 78%, then the Zone group with 77%, and then the Learn group with 76% retention. For reference, the Ornish diet is a very low fat (10% of energy as fat) diet, high in carbohydrates.

Besides, I don't think the A to Z study is really reflective of the nature of what I am trying to say here. Judging by the composition of their macronutrient intake, Gardner [59] reports that the Atkins group was eating: 17-32% carbohydrates, 22-28% protein, and 46-55% fat from the total caloric intake. Remember that Phinney and Volek [5] consider a high-fat diet one that starts at 60% fat from total calories and 5-10% carbohydrates from the total calories.

If most of the people on the Atkins diet follow similar nutrient partitioning as Gardner [59] did in his 1 year study, and if they have such great results, then I ask you:

What do you think happens when you go further on lowering the carbohydrate intake and increasing the fat intake?

Again, there are not too many good studies including well formulated high-fat diets. This is why many proponents of high-carb diets dismiss the well formulated ketogenic studies. It's also because there are very few subjects recruited in these types of studies. However, I'm very positive that things are changing and that more good science is to come in the following years. I will do my best into trying to further this cause.

Cholesterol and Lipoproteins

Ever since the low-fat dogma has started circulating throughout the world, cholesterol has become some sort of public enemy number 1. Yet, very few people know that cholesterol and phospholipids are essential to normal life and that they are found in almost all the cells of our body.

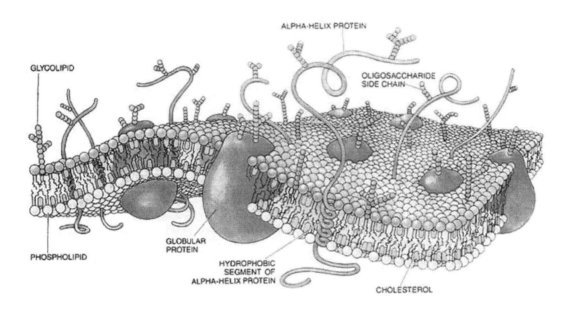

We know that all cells are surrounded by a membrane [60]. This membrane is predominant in phospholipids as you can see in the image above. These phospholipids make up the lipid bilayer of the membrane. One can observe the cholesterol droplets that are inside the lipid membrane. We could not function if the mechanisms producing phospholipids and cholesterol for all membranes are deficient. The same goes for the brain, which is approximately 60% fat [61].

According to Chang, Ke, and Chen [61], fatty acids are among the most important molecules in determining human brain integrity. They consider that EFA (essential fatty acids) are needed to sustain a good state of health and that they cannot be synthesized by the body, which is why they have to enter the body by ingestion (eating fat). They reference studies that have related to impaired brain performance correlated to imbalanced dietary fat intake.

It's no wonder that I feel more mentally equipped ever since I started eating high-fat-very-low-carb. Again, it may be just me but I have an inclination for doing complex brain tasks. An example would be that I developed a passion for studying the human metabolism and the human brain. If it weren't for this ketogenic lifestyle, I wouldn't have been writing this book now.

Even though Chang, Ke, and Chen [61] say that the body is not able to synthesize all the essential fatty acids it needs for good health, I know there are studies pointing out that little of the cholesterol that is ingested has an impact on blood cholesterol levels. Peter Attia considers that roughly 25% of the total cholesterol we have in our bodies is from what we eat, while the rest of 75% is synthesized by the human body [62].

If you can take a quick look at my blood samples after two months of high-fat nutrition (68-75% of total calories as fat), you can see that my total cholesterol has increased [63]. When I started the experiment, I was not wise enough to measure anything other than total cholesterol. I didn't know much about lipids, lipoproteins, and cholesterol back then.

At Day 0 of the experiment - 19.09.2013 - the total cholesterol was 162 mg/dL. So I had "normal" total cholesterol values (lower than 200 mg/dL) and I was on track. However, I did not know how much of it was TAG (triglycerides), how much of it was HDL-C, and how much of it was LDL-C.

Two months later - 12.12.2013 - my total cholesterol measured 217 mg/dL. The general guidelines would say I had high-cholesterol levels, but let's examine the facts. After two months of constant reading and lecturing on the human metabolism, I was a little wiser and measured the other markers mentioned above. I measured the triglycerides levels and they were 40 mg/dL, in the context in which normal triglycerides values are < 150mg/dL.

My LDL cholesterol was 124 mg/dL, while the normal values required it to be below 130mg/dL (so, it's okay). My HDL cholesterol was 77.7 mg/dL in the context in which values higher than 35 mg/dL are considered normal. Triglycerides have increased to 74 mg/dL; however, they were still way below the 150 mg/dL risk level.

So, if you take a look at all these lipid biomarkers, they were all in the normal range, but the total cholesterol was higher than "normal", showing 217 mg/dL. But, how is total cholesterol measured?

Total Cholesterol = LDLc + HDLc + TAG/5

Let's fill in with my biomarkers from December 2013:

Total Cholesterol = 124 + 77.7 + 74/5

Total Cholesterol = 216.5 mg/dL

If there could only be a way to measure HDLc and LDLc by only knowing Total Cholesterol and TAG, now I would know the values of these two by plugging-in the data from the beginning of my experiment in late September.

I'm pretty positive there are ways to approximate these particles only by knowing TC and TAG, but I have not been curious enough so far to find them.

So, as long as each of the biomarkers are within a good range of values, I would not worry what the Total Cholesterol formula shows. The key take away in this case is that the cholesterol ingested has a little contribution to body's total cholesterol because our bodies create most of the cholesterol they need. Besides, only about 20% of the cholesterol that is synthesized is created in the liver, while the rest of 80% is synthesized by the cells [64].

I could go further more into the details talking about lipoproteins. It is an extremely interesting subject to see how the fats ingested are taken from the intestines and delivered to the liver and to other parts in the body. However, I can spare you some time and invite you to view this amazingly interactive video that explains Lipoproteins, Apolipoproteins, and Familial Dyslipidemias [65]. The key take-away is that when you restrict carbohydrates and increase fat intake, your lipid profile improves, a.k.a. all lipid biomarkers show better values.

Dr. Stephen Sinatra is a great heart physicians who has well documented the role that cholesterol has in the human body, the correlation between saturated fatty acids and heart disease, as well as in research having to do with grounding (the idea that going bare-feet on the ground - being connected to Mother Earth) supports an exchange of electrons between the human body and the earth that leads to lower oxidative damage to the body and lower utilization of ATP for energy production). For starters, just read Dr. Sinatra's book *The Great Cholesterol Myth* [66].

Inflammation and Reactive Oxygen Species

This chapter is the most extensive so far because it has to do with the health implications that ketogenic nutrition has on the human body. There have been proponents of high-carbohydrate nutrition that tell me something like this:

"Oh, yes...Ketogenic diets are good in treating diseases and different health issues, but they should not be followed by normal healthy individuals."

Again, my logic, even as biased as it is right now, makes me think:

How something that saves you from major health issues cannot be good to follow on a daily basis?

What's the rationale behind the fact that you should use ketogenic diets to treat different health conditions and jump back to a normal carb-ish diet when your health improves?

Is this flawed or is it just me being flawed?

The next point that I want to touch upon is inflammation. This is a subject that I didn't give too much attention up until I was very familiar with ketogenic nutrition. Even though I would like to keep things as simple as possible, researching to write this part of the book makes me reconsider the higher importance that inflammation and reactive oxygen species (oxidative stress) have on our lives.

If we can maintain inflammation at lower levels inside our bodies we will not only improve the quality of our lives, but we will also increase our lifespan. Many of the diseases that grow to become epidemics nowadays have inflammation as their root causes. Phinney and Volek [5] have a simple definition of inflammation:

"Inflammation is part of what we sometimes call immunity or host defense. It is that complex mix of functions that our bodies use to defend against foreign substances and infections, and also how it stimulates the healing process after injury."

So, inflammation is good in our bodies, at very low levels because it helps us fight infections and it keeps our bodies protected. There are various biomarkers which reflect the level of inflammation in the human body, such: C reactive protein and Interleukin (CRP and IL-6). You can find out these levels when doing a simple blood work.

It would be fair to discuss inflammation in the context of reactive oxygen species. If you look into biochemistry textbooks, there may not be too much information about oxidative stress, ROS (reactive oxygen species) and inflammation. Or, at least I was not able to find decent information.

According to Held [67], reactive oxygen species are reactive molecules and free radicals derived from molecular oxygen. They play a key role in cell signaling and in the activation of cell signaling cascades. They are important when it comes to apoptosis (programmed cell death), as well as gene expression. They can be: superoxide, hydrogen peroxide, hydroxyl radical, nitric oxide, and hydroxyl ion (image courtesy [67]):

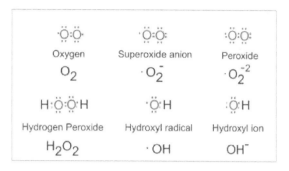

Figure 1. Electron structures of common reactive oxygen species. Each structure is provided with its name and chemical formula. The t designates an unpaired electron.

The major source of ROS production is mitochondrial respiration.

Whoaw. Wait. **What's a mitochondrion?** (image courtesy [69])

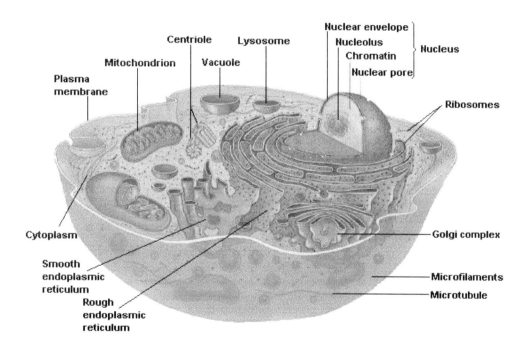

Mitochondria are the powerhouses of the cells, without which we would not be able to get the energy from the nutrients and use it for cellular functions throughout the body [70]. So, the mitochondrion is the place where all the magic happens.

There is a part in the mitochondria called the electron transport chain (ETC) and this is the site where most ROS are produced. Even at this point I think I went into too much detail and I would not want to stress you out. If there are biochemistry freaks who want to dig into details, you can check this one out [71].

The production of ROS in the mitochondria and also in the endoplasmic reticulum can contribute to the aging process as well as to the development of diseases such as Parkinson and T2D, as well as other degenerative diseases. (image courtesy of [72])

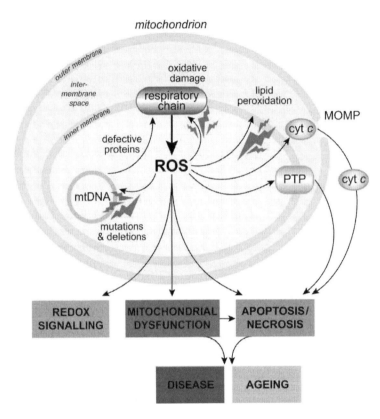

Murphy [72] reports that oxidative damage can be reached by broken ROS production by mitochondria and this can result in impaired ability to produce ATP (energy currency of the body), damage to mitochondrial membranes and DNA, and damage to various functions of the mitochondria.

I must admit that at this point in my life, my thinking is pretty much biased. I am now biased because I tend to view the many positive things that happen as I follow this type of lifestyle. There have been so many benefits of the ketogenic lifestyle on my quality of life that I firmly believe that it could benefit many people.

Of course, my approach is a bit different because unlike other people, I have not experienced hormonal dis-regulation and I was able to increase my muscle mass slightly, as well as my physical performance, both in strength training and in endurance exercise. I would not completely attribute this to nutrition alone, but I think there are a couple of factors why this worked great for me and I think that cold thermogenesis is one of them.

I will talk a lot more about these factors in the chapter dedicated to performance, but I just wanted to touch upon this because I think that like myself, there are many others with biased thinking. :)

On the other side, I like to objectively analyze the data from my life and try to see if implemented within the same boundaries would be of service to others as well. So, let's talk a bit about good science and bad science and ROS.

Remember I have already told you about these proponents of high-carbohydrate diets and the way in which "bad" studies are conducted. Many researchers see high-fat diets as diets consisting of 35-55% fat, and 30-40% carbs, while the rest is protein. Whenever doing research studies under these conditions, the results are poor (to say the least).

They put a big burden onto the shoulders of high-fat nutrition. Besides, there are other researchers who want to do things better, so they follow a good high fat diet according to macronutrient partitioning as follows: 60+% of calories as fat, 5-10% of calories as carbohydrates, and the rest of the calories as protein from the total daily intake of energy.

However, the flaw in this approach is the limited amount of time they conduct this type of research. Most of the studies conducted under these parameters have lasted somewhere from 1 day to 5-6 days. Most of you know that this is insufficient time to become fat adapted. Hence, the poor results of these experiments tend to produce a bias against a well formulated high-fat diet.

To accentuate this point, let's dig a bit into this research study from 2012 [73]. It is entitled *Age and High Fat Diet Associated Changes in Mitochondrial ROS Production in the Liver.* It was conducted at Munich University by several researchers. Their hypothesis was that a high-fat diet will lead to deposition of fat in tissues which will lead to impaired insulin signaling as well as modifications in the mitochondrial output.

The so called bad experiments that I am referring to do not even bother to explain the macronutrient partitioning they have used. Some of them do. This study did as well. So, they call a high-fat diet as one that has 45% of the total caloric intake as fat, 35% of the total caloric intake as carbohydrates, and 18% of the total caloric intake as protein. The control group was eating 12% of the total caloric intake as fat, 65% of the total caloric intake as carbohydrates, and ~23% of the total caloric intake as protein. To make matters worse, fat sources in the diet were soy oil and palm oil for the high-fat group and soy-oil for the control group. The studies were conducted on mice.

So, the general inexperienced reader who does not know what a well formulated high-fat-very-low-carbohydrate diet is, would believe these types of research studies as being well designed, hence they will promote the "fat is bad" message.

Here's another research study that I suspect to be of the same kind. I was not able to access the full version which is why I say "I suspect" it has been designed with the same "high-fat" protocol as the previous one. This study [74] was done on rats and it started from the hypothesis that a high-fat diet affects liver metabolism, it leads to insulin resistance, and mitochondrial alterations.

They put rats on an 8 week high-fat diet and they concluded that this type of nutrition results in profound mitochondrial lipid composition. They also saw an inhibition in fatty acid oxidation, as well as a higher ROS production. I would really like to see the composition of this high-fat diet.

On the other end of the spectrum, let's examine the research studies conducted on well formulated ketogenic diets. This study [75] was done on mice and it is entitled "*The Ketogenic Diet Reverses Gene Expression Patterns and Reduces Reactive Oxygen Species Levels when used as an Adjuvant Therapy for Glioma*". They compared the patterns of gene expression in tumors vs. normal brains from animals that were fed either a high-fat ketogenic diet or a standard diet.

In this case the high fat diet consisted of 8.36% of the total caloric intake as proteins, .76% (?) of the total caloric intake as carbohydrates and 78.8% of the total caloric intake as fat. They were being supplied with vitamins and minerals. The researchers observed that the ketogenic diet improved survivability in the mouse model and that it reduced ROS production in tumor cells. Another study [76] shows just about the same results saying that "ketones inhibit mitochondrial production of ROS following glutamate excitotoxicity by increasing NADH oxidation".

Let's move on to research studies conducted on humans. Here is a study [77] done on subjects consuming high-carbohydrate vs. high-fat meals. The study followed inflammation and reactive oxidative stress responses to these diets in healthy humans.

It was done on 15 healthy individuals (drawback: lower number of subjects) and it analyzed their response to either of the diets (high-fat vs. high-carb) after 1000 kcals meals. This may be another drawback over the high-fat part of the study because the subjects may have not been keto-adapted. It takes weeks to keto-adapt so giving a person who is not keto-adapted a high-fat meal will make him/her react differently compared to giving the same meal to a keto-adapted individual.

They analyzed the expression of IL6, IL8, and plasma total antioxidative status 3 hours after the meal. They've seen increase in IL6 regardless of the diet, lower IL18 on the high-fat diet, and they concluded that a high-carb meal can evoke a greater post-prandial oxidative stress response.

I think this study is reflective of its purpose because the researchers wanted to determine the effects of two different meal approaches on inflammation and oxidative stress response. However, I'm very curios to see the results and responses in a similar study where keto-adapted persons are compared with people consuming high-carbohydrate diets.

Another study [78] which appeared in *Nutrition and Metabolism* in 2008 followed the inflammatory response to carbohydrate restricted diets in overweight men. They gathered 28 overweight men and put them on carbohydrate restricted diets where their total caloric intake was: 17% carbohydrates, 57% fat, and 26% protein.

The unique aspect of this study was that the diet required the subjects to eat lots of eggs (640mg of additional cholesterol/day coming from eggs). 15 men were being assigned this type of egg consumption while the other 13 men were the placebo group and they did not consume additional dietary cholesterol. The study lasted for 12 weeks.

Although I would have liked to see this study modified where the subjects had more calories coming from fat (60+%) and fewer from carbohydrates (<10%), the results were as follows: lower body fat for all subjects, higher adiponectin (involved in the regulation of fatty acid oxidation glucose levels. - higher is better), lower CRP in the group consuming many eggs (C-Reactive Protein - biomarker of inflammation), MCP-1 levels were lower for the group not consuming eggs and unchanged in the group consuming many eggs. Other inflammation biomarkers were not affected by the diet and/or by the egg consumption.

Researchers have concluded that carbohydrate restricted diets associated with increased egg consumption lowers inflammation probably because of the effect of higher HDL-C ("good" cholesterol) and to the antioxidant lutein which regulates different inflammatory responses. Alrighty, now let me just go and grab some dozen eggs.

Phinney and Volek [5] give a fair explanation of very low carbohydrate diets and their impact on inflammation. They cite studies that show how low-carb diets reduce inflammation and how many of these subjects show lower levels of CRP and IL6. They also caution on the effect of higher inflammation that leads to the subsequent development of the metabolic syndrome. Their bottom line is that "a host of biomarkers of inflammation (known inducers of ROS generation) go down when a low carb diet is adopted." [5].

One personal story that I'd like to share on this topic is that before adopting the ketogenic lifestyle I was getting pimples and acne on my neck after shaving. Some of them would stay there for months and my skin was becoming swollen and ached. It was pretty uncomfortable.

One month after starting the ketogenic nutrition it was all gone and it hasn't appeared since. As an added bonus, I do not need to use after-shave lotions and gels to prevent skin irritation after shaving. I find this to be very beneficial.

In the end of this section, I want to point out the importance of good research studies. To avoid biased thinking it is good to try and see several ends of the spectrum, as well as the middle portion of the spectrum. I want to draw the attention on what well formulated high-fat ketogenic diets are, as well as on what so called high-fat (high-fat-high-carb) diets are. Make sure you have this in mind whenever you are reading research on the topic.

Further readings on the subject should include Dr. Jack Kruse's blog and book *The Epi-Paleo Rx*. Among others he's presented compelling research on EMF radiation and it's negative effects on the human body, as well as on how to increase the Redox potential, hence promoting optimal health and increasing life-span.

Seizures, Alzheimer's, Parkinson's Disease, and Cancer Therapy

This is an amplification of the previously discussed subject. Basically, many of the health issues from the title have a certain degree of correlation with inflammation. For a better understanding of each one of them, they should briefly be defined.

Seizures occur when abnormal signals from the brain affect the way in which the body behaves. They can be associated with high electrical activity inside the brain. Epilepsy is characterized by the occurrence of seizures as a result of contributing factors like malignancies, trauma and infections which are accompanied by CNS (central nervous system) inflammation [79].

Alzheimer disease is a mental issue which is characterized by dementia and failing memory. There are various other manifestations in AD, such as: poor judgment, confusion, hallucinations, agitation, increased muscle tone (occasionally), seizures (occasionally), and others. This is a degenerative disease that typically lasts for 8 to 10 years [80].

Alzheimer's occurs when plaques and tangles (two abnormal proteins) accumulate and kill brain cells. It all starts in the hippocampus (the region of the brain where memory is formed) and it spreads out throughout the brain destroying different regions and impairing the person suffering from this disease (image courtesy of American Health Assistance Foundation).

Normal Brain vs. Alzheimer's Patient Brain

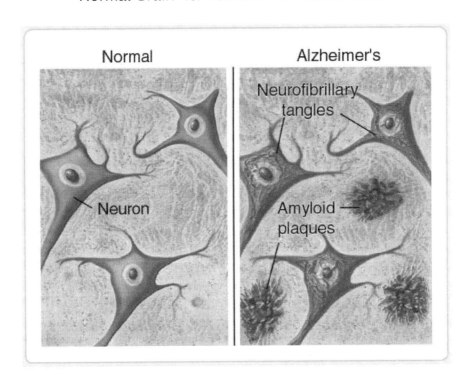

Alzheimer's Disease spreads to the language area of the brain, then to the area of the brain where logic is, then to the emotional area, then to the sensory cortex (where the processing of input from sensory organs occur), then to the back of the brain (which is involved with long-term memory), ultimately affecting parts of the brain regulating un-conditioned reflexes such as heart beats and breathing.

Moving on to **Parkinson's Disease**, the simplest way to explain it is that it is characterized by a diminished release of dopamine in the Substantia Nigra area of the brain. Dopamine is a neurotransmitter released in synapses. When there is a shortage of dopamine, there will be less of it in the synapses, and this ultimately leads to motor, cognitive, and behavioral deficits.

Cancer can simply be explained by an abnormal growth of cells. We have approximately 30-40 trillion cells in the human body [81]. At every second some of them replicate and create new cells while older versions of those cells die off (through a process called apoptosis - programmed cell death) and not only. Various factors (genetic, environmental and nutritional to name a few) can lead to dysfunctions in this process of programmed cell death so that the cells replicate uncontrollably. This is how cancer tumors are created. They can either be localized (in a specific location) or metastasized (spread throughout the body).

Neurological disorders have been shown to have inflammation as one of their root causes and also as a contributing factor to the progression of these disorders. This study from 2013 [79] says that data collected from experimental models of epilepsy as well as from human brain tissue support the fact that inflammation is involved in seizures. IL-1 beta, TNF (tumor necrosis factor), and IL-6 are some of the key mediators of this process.

Another study [82] starts on the premise that oxidative stress which results from excessive release of free radicals can be very much involved in the initiation and progression of epilepsy, which is why anti-oxidants and therapies involving them have been given special attention in treating seizures and epilepsy. I wonder why they don't focus on limiting the oxidative stress resulting rather than trying to reduce the damage afterwards.

Why focus on the symptoms instead of treating the causes?

Very recent research [83] brings into discussion the accumulation of toxic protein in mitochondria which results in energy deficits, higher reactive oxygen species generation, mutations, and impaired mitochondrial output both in animal models and in patients of neurodegenerative diseases, such as Parkinson's disease.

One study that caught my attention was this one from December 2013 [84]. It starts on the premise that inflammation occurs in neurodegenerative diseases such as Parkinson, Alzheimer, Huntington, as well as amyotrophic lateral sclerosis. The researchers highlight the importance of establishing different biomarkers of inflammation that would easily be measurable "reproducible, not subject to wide variation in the population, and unaffected by external factors". So, they are basically taking inflammation for granted and they want to select a few biomarkers that could be used efficiently in preventing and, most likely, in treating these conditions.

I will not give specific case studies of how ketogenic diets have efficiently been used in reducing and controlling seizures and epileptic episodes ever since the early 1900s. The research on this subject is overwhelming. If you browse the medical databases you will find tons of examples.

However, I'm intrigued by the fact that it still is not promoted as a very important and primary tool for seizures. It is considered to be difficult to maintain. However, I would rather go with a dietary approach in treating a certain disorder rather than going on drugs or other more invasive and potentially dangerous treatments. Besides, there are few good physicians who can formulate appropriate ketogenic diets for epileptic patients.

These types of ketogenic diets are extremely high in fat (90% fat from total calories) and very low in carbohydrates. Also, they are very efficient if they are hypocaloric as well. A good book on this subject is the one written by Kossoff, Freeman, Zahava, and Rubenstein in 2011 entitled *Ketogenic Diets: Treatments for Epilepsy and Other Disorders* [85].

Ketogenic diets are very efficient in combating these neurodegenerative diseases mostly because of the effect that ketone bodies has on energy metabolism inside the brain. They have been shown to produce fewer reactive oxygen species, thus lower oxidative stress.

There is the incredible research and story of Dr. Mary Newport whose husband was suffering from Alzheimer's and his condition was deteriorating progressively at a faster pace. Approximately 3 or 4 years into the disease, Mary discovered medium-chain triglycerides in the form of coconut oil and started administering her husband several teaspoons of it per day.

His condition improved rapidly: from being unable to do simple math computations, from being unable to recognize family members, from getting lost, from having language and communication problems, and from not knowing how to open the refrigerator, to being able to read after a few months on MCT oil intake, then to being able to use the lawn-mower to cut the grass and to overall improve his health condition [86].

Mary was so thrilled of the improvements she saw with her husband that tried to advocate for the usage of MCTs in Alzheimer's patients but she was never able to get very far due to the rejections and resistance she experienced from well established institutions such as the Alzheimer's Associations, Dr. Oz, Oprah, and even a Supreme Court Justice member. However, she didn't give up and conducted a small research on her own. She started getting in contact with care givers of people suffering from Alzheimer's. Here's her published results (image courtesy of [86]:

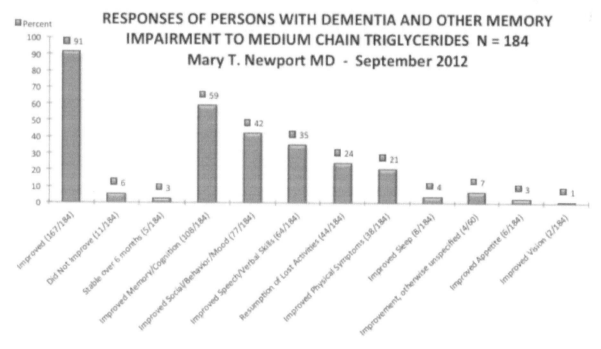

I find these results very promising. I know further research is required, but we know at least a direction has been established. I am also interested into conducting more research on the implications of ketogenic approaches to Parkinson's disease patients, as there is not too much data on this. Also, there is not much research on dietary approaches for these neuro-degenerative diseases, besides epilepsy (which is not advocated by medical institutions, sadly).

In terms of cancer therapy, this dietary intervention may have huge potential. I am pretty sure of that. However, at the current moment most of the surgeons, medical doctors, and other types of practitioners are not even aware of the implications of nutrients in correlation with cancer development and growth.

Remember that I've told you about the cancer cells and their dysfunctions. One of the dysfunction is that they do not know when to die, so they replicate abnormally. Another dysfunction has a lot to do with metabolism. Now, let's talk about the Warburg Effect. The best way to understand it would be through an illustration (image courtesy of [88]).

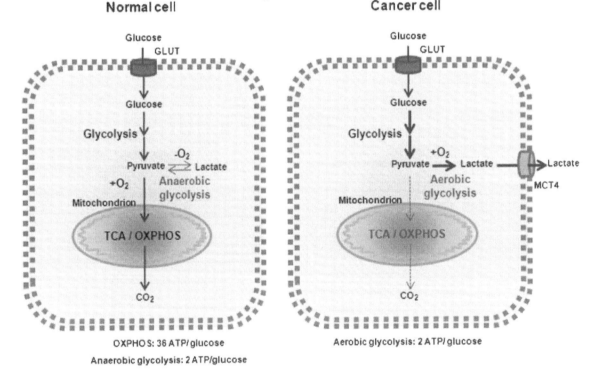

There is a metabolic difference between normal cells and cancer cells. Normal cells will turn glucose into pyruvate for survival and growth and then they will fully oxidize pyruvate to carbon dioxide through the Krebs (TCA) Cycle and through Oxidative Phosphorylation. The net energy yield of this process is approximately 34-36 ATPs for a molecule of glucose. This process is oxygen dependent [88].

On the other hand, when there is a shortage of oxygen, pyruvate will be turned to lactate. Cancer cells will turn most of the glucose coming-in to lactate, no matter how much oxygen is available. This is called the Warburg Effect. When this happens and more glucose is diverted to lactate (anabolic processes), less energy will be produced (because pyruvate does not enter the TCA cycle) and this will accelerate cell proliferation (multiplication and growth). Less energy is produced (approximately 2 molecules of ATP per molecule of glucose) [87].

Now you should understand cancer more than most people. The next thing that you need to know is that while the majority of the cells in the human body can switch to using ketone bodies for energy generation, cancer cells (luckily) do not have this ability. At least many of them don't.

This means that cancer cells can't utilize beta-oxidation efficiently. Up until now, we know that many forms of cancer are glucose dependent. The Warburg Effect is an explanation of this. Besides, how do you think that cancer tumors are being spotted?

Cancer tumors are localized through FDG-PET Scans. FDG stands for fluoro-2-deoxy-glucose. PET (Positron Emission Tomography) scans use small amounts of radioactive tracers that are injected in the patients' body to expose the differences between healthy and diseased tissues.

In FDG-PET Scans, a certain amount of FDG is injected into the patient. Since it is glucose based, it will be up-taken by the cells. But normal cells will show a slower and more reduced uptake compared to cancer cells, which will absorb more of it faster. The PET scanner will detect the radiation coming from the FDG in the body and will show the areas where FDG concentration is increased [89].

The key take-away that you should know is that many types of cancer cells consume much more glucose than normal cells and they go into anaerobic metabolism. Again, while the majority of the cells in the human body can adapt to using ketones to produce energy, cancer cells do not have this ability. Hence, if you starve the body of glucose, cancer cells will most likely die off.

There are folks who reject this approach. Many physicians are not even aware of such thing and the research is just starting to become decently substantial. A lot of work that has been done and it is currently ongoing in this field is conducted by Dominic D'Agostino, an Assistant Professor at the University of South Florida, Department of Molecular Pharmacology and Physiology.

Besides cancer research, Dominic has been working with Navy Seals analyzing the effects of ketogenic nutrition on their physiologies. He's also been studying ketogenic diets in the context of brain disorders and oxidative stress. Some of the research and work done and "to be completed" by Dominic D'Agostino are found here [90].

I could not end this chapter without referring to one of the greatest door openers in the field of cancer research, Thomas Seyfried. D'Agostino and Seyfried both have done different research studies together. Thomas Seyfried has an amazing book called *Cancer as a Metabolic Disease: On the Origin, Management, and Prevention of Cancer* [91]. It's basically based upon the nutritional approach to treating cancer.

One thing that I do not like about Seyfried (maybe it's just me) is that he doesn't do what he preaches. He's written a book on ketogenic diets and cancer, but I've listened to an interview of him where he said that he was not particularly following a ketogenic diet. Again, this is only my opinion and it should stay that way. Seyfried has done amazing work in the field of cancer research and he should be praised for that.

This was quite a long chapter and hopefully you are now very well familiar with all the health concepts and implications of very-low-carbohydrate-high-fat nutrition. In the next chapter I will talk about physical performance under this protocol.

Chapter Six

Ketoadaptation: Strength, Endurance and Physical Performance

What they say

If you are into sports, either for performance or just for recreation, you may have heard multiple times that ketogenic diets are detrimental to increasing muscle mass. Some also say they have experienced negative effects on their endurance training. But isn't this message of the same kind with what you're hearing in the media or on TV?

The general guidelines still promote very high-carbohydrate diets even though they were proven to be bad for our health. The media is still promoting the same "avoid salt, sugar, and saturated fats" message, which is only partially applicable.

If you go to your local gym and if you know something about proper training, nutrition, and rest, you will get a major headache. Almost everyone is doing it wrong (according to my biased thinking and their visual appearance).

I see people working out by doing many sets with many repetitions for strength training. I see them doing the repetitions the wrong way and the result they will get is totally different from expectations. I feel frustrated and sometimes angry because I've seen many people attending gyms for a long time with no visible results. I know people staying in the gym for more than 2 hours everyday or every 2 days with no improvements in their physical shape and performance.

The gyms have become places for socialization and marketing places for protein shakes and supplements. This only serves to reinforce my biases.

I know many people who workout and drink protein shakes before, after, and even during training. Then they take energy drinks (I did it as well), then they take creatine, glutamine (guilty as charged), and then they take all sorts of pills that allegedly will "help" them become physically better.

Yet, these supplements taken by people without any knowledge of proper nutrition and exercise will never serve their purpose. Please do not get me wrong because I believe that we are not able to get all the proper nutrients from our nutrition alone or if this was the case, we would have to eat huge amounts of a specific food just to get a certain substance into our body (for example Omega-3 fatty acids - I'll talk about them in a later chapter).

Bad nutrition combined with bad exercise (overtraining) will cause much more harm than good. If you're just starting going to the gym or working out, the basic rule that I would recommend is:

Take advice only from the people who do what they preach. Take advice from the people who show that their protocols have been working for them. Translation:

All of us "know" what one has to do to lose weight and to become healthier. Even the fat person next to you will tell you that you have to do this and that so that you can become this or that. Only listen (don't act upon) to what they're saying *if they really act and show results upon what they are saying*.

Let me give you a quick example:

Since I travel a lot, I do not pay for monthly subscriptions to gyms. I just pay per session. I've been into many gyms so far. A few days ago, I went to a new gym and the first thing I did was to map the place. Not being able to find the chest press machine, I politely asked the personal trainer:

Me: Excuse me, please tell me where the chest press machine is.
Him: What do you want to do?
Me: I just need to find the chest press, please.
Him: What particular muscle you want to work out? We can go for the upper chest or lower chest. There's no chest press that efficiently works

out the entire chest. Come with me. We can do the chest press with the barbell, or you can try this one.....

In my mind: Really dude, wtf? I was asking you to point out where the chest press is. It is simple: yes or no. Don't give me the full history of strength training and the types of exercises I wanna do. I know what I want. (me over-reacting!)

He noticed the fact that I was kind of irritated by his response and he saw that I was clear on what I wanted to do, unlike many of the people that are confused in the gym and follow everything without question. So, he left me alone.

Please excuse me for being judgmental but that particular personal trainer was not entitled to give me advice because he was nowhere near what I would call a "good physical condition". He was "fluffy" and his belly fat was more than observable.

Since I couldn't find the machine I was looking for, I combined two different presses to get a good chest workout.

The key take away on this is that before going to a gym and being dragged into doing something that you wouldn't like to do or wouldn't be good for you, do your homework. Know exactly what you want to accomplish (build muscle, lose fat, both?) and start looking for the best online resources you can find on the topic. Look for experts in these areas and don't rely on just one.

Delve into what many experts have to say about a certain topic and try to reach a conclusion based upon your research. Once you have this knowledge at hand, you can start walking in the gym or on the jogging track with confidence and with little chance of having someone push something bad down your throat.

Another thing that I want to say before getting deeper into the science is: once you do your own research, make sure you learn how to do the exercises correctly (I'm emphasizing this because many people and personal-trainers do them incorrectly). Being well informed will keep you away from getting hurt.

Besides, you don't have to carry a 2L water bottle with you all the time and have a mouthful after each repetition. Do your own research on this and if you are thorough, you'll draw the same conclusion. You don't need that much water for 30 minutes to an hour of training. Yet, most of the people inside the gym carry their water bottles and protein shakes like they were stranded in the desert.

There are so many bad practices around that I do not even know where to start. From my research and from my personal experience, I find that almost everything that I see happening in the gym and in the nutrition field is bad practice. You need to stay away from that.

We have to touch upon these points from various perspectives:

1. Nutrition - common beliefs vs. the science of ketogenic nutrition for higher physical performance

2. Exercise - common beliefs and practices vs. science + experience of experts over decades

3. Resting (period of no-exercise) - common beliefs and practices vs. science

I will try to integrate my humble experience and practices along the way.

Nutrition and Performance for the Keto-adapted Endurance Trainee

I'm not sure if you know what most people eat and drink during marathons, Ironman challenges, and other ultra endurance training. There is a billion dollar industry behind nutrition for the ultra-athlete. You should know that most of the athletes who participate in such competitions follow a normal diet (which tends to be low-fat and high-carbohydrate).

Let's take for example a marathon which is ~42km of running. During a marathon, there are re-feeding points where the runners can have foods (on the go) that would provide them with readily available energy to be burned (sugary foods - bars, chocolate, bananas, etc). Also, many athletes carry around different gels and drinks that are carbohydrate-rich and can be taken on the go..

You know that I've told you about our glucose tank of ~2000kcals (at maximum). This is the amount of energy that we can save in our glycogen stores (as carbohydrates). Once the carbohydrate tank is depleted, an athlete's body urgently demands more readily available energy.

This explains the phenomena of "hitting the wall". When you start running low on glucose (in the context of high-carb burners), your brain starts experiencing "panic", you want to give up, and you feel that your feet are letting you down. If glycogen stores go too low, your brain can simply just turn-off your muscles and you become exhausted. Hitting the wall is a condition experienced by many athletes and it is associated with symptoms like fatigue, general weakness, lower motivation, foggy mind (dizziness) and sometimes even hallucinations.

Okay, I guess you already know about this situation because it has been discussed all over the online. I find it very interesting because once you start questioning general beliefs and try to go further into the science and the research, you start seeing how one moves slowly away from the dogma into a totally different zone.

Most athletes attending these competitions do not know there is another approach (at least one) and if you start saying something different to them, they tell you that it is non-sense and that there is no science behind what you are saying. Now, let me explain.

In October 2013, a few weeks after going full keto, I met an old friend while walking down the street. I barely recognized him. I was more or less shocked. When I saw him a year before he told me he wanted to start going to the gym (because he wanted to improve his physical condition and lose the extra pounds).

At that time, he was more than overweight. He was moderately obese. Now, he was this thin guy, hence my reaction! So, I told him that we should get together and chat for a while. A couple of days later we met and he told me the whole story.

Basically, he went to a local gym, got an instructor, and got some "sport nutrition" products. He discovered the products of this company (world-wide giant) and along with the low-intensity prolonged training he was able to lose approximately 50 kg (~120 pounds) in a matter of months.

This company, let's call it X-Nutrition, builds cults in every big city in the world. If you become a promoter of X-Nutrition products, you get discounts for these products, you get the support of the local community, and you also get trained to be a promoter.

It is like an MLM company. They attract people into buying their products and becoming their promoters by offering free consultations and body composition assessments. I was very curious and took the free consultation because I wanted to see how they are trained and what they are going to tell me about my nutrition and what they are going to suggest me I do to increase my physical performance.

I wasn't surprised to find out that they are poorly trained. The person who assessed me told me that to increase my lean mass I have to eat 4-6 meals a day, that I do not have to skip breakfast, and that I have to eat 30g of protein per meal because my body cannot efficiently use more than this amount. Why 30g? Why not 31g? Why not 29? Is that specific amount of 30g imprinted into our DNA?

I tended to believe that person until I started researching this claim and started experimenting on my own. For example, this study [92] shows that feeding approximately 80% of the recommended daily protein intake in one meal had no difference compared to feeding it in 4 meals spread throughout the day. The study follows 16 women over a period of 14 days and the researchers conclude there is no statistical difference between the groups in terms of protein absorption and degradation.

Another study [93] followed intermittent fasters who only ate in a 4 hour window every day. They had to have all their meals (and energy intake) during these four hours. The 4 hours were followed by 20 hours of fasting. This means that they would have to go much over the 30g prescription in 4 hours in terms of protein intake. The researchers wanted to see the body composition changes and had concluded that this type of nutrition and feeding pattern did not affect muscle preservation.

So, is 30g a myth? I tend to believe so, but it needs further research because these two studies that I easily located are not enough to give a strong conclusion. I personally eat more than 30g of protein per meal (in ketosis) and I did not find any impact on me in a negative way (so far).

I may have gotten far from my point but I wanted to focus on the fact that those promoters from the nutrition company were not being taught well and they transmitted the same flawed messages. They said that I need a good source of pure protein that is not part of my meals and that I should buy one of their products.

My friend who lost ~50kg is a promoter of those products and he claims that he could not do long-runs without carrying some gels (rich in carbs) and some high-protein-high-carb bars with him all the time.

Again, I want to reemphasize that you should do your own research before following a particular dogma which can possibly be flawed. Read articles and read other people's experiences on the subject. Most importantly, follow the opinions of the experts and find research studies (Google Scholar or The PubMed Library are a good start) to verify their claims.

Another side of the coin is when fat-adapted athletes are running in ultra-endurance competitions. When one is adapted to burning fat as a primary source of fuel, carbohydrates are less relevant (and needed). The brain does not go into panic mode, the motivation levels are higher, fatigue is less present, and recovery usually happens quicker.

A keto-adapted athlete can run an entire marathon or even further by only carrying some water with him. The fat tank that each one of us has on their body is much (20 times, at least) greater than the glycogen tank. Even lean athletes (4-5% body fat) have at least 35,000-40,000 kcals stored as bodyfat [2].

A normal weight person of 80kg (180 pounds) will burn ~3000kcals during a marathon [94]. Since your fat tank is at least 12 times larger than that, you could easily run a marathon using nothing but your own body fat. How cool is that!? There are several examples of fat adapted athletes, such Ben Greenfield [95] or Tim Olsen [96] to name a few.

The best part of going into ultra-endurance challenges while being keto-adapted is that you don't feel exhausted at the end of the competition compared to how you feel if you burned carbohydrates for fuel.

Another benefit is that you can now burn the stubborn fat from your body because if you run and you are on high-carb nutrition, there is a very small likelihood you would efficiently and substantially use body fat for energy.

A high-carb burner who runs marathons can oxidize little fat for energy, given that he depends on carbohydrates. However, Jeff Volek [96] and Peter Attia [2] have shown that keto-adapted athletes can derive more than 90% of their energy needs from fat during ultra-endurance events. This means you're running almost entirely on fat. Again, how cool is that!

There have been various good studies conducted on very low-carbohydrate athletes but they have not been credited throughout the literature. Again, it seems like the folks are ignoring the data. Ever since the 1980s, Steve Phinney [5] did research on keto-adapted cyclists who showed no reduction in their performance after a period of adaptation of several weeks. Let's see what the research was about.

This study [97] appeared in *Metabolism* in 1983 and it was conducted by Stephen Phinney and four other researchers. They wanted to determine the human metabolic response to chronic ketosis without caloric restriction. They studied 5 well trained cyclists for 5 weeks. The first week they were being fed with a eucaloric balanced diet (EBD) consisting of 1.75g protein/kg per day and the remaining calories were 2/3 carbohydrates and 1/3 fat. So it was a high-carbohydrate diet.

Then, they fed the athletes with a eucaloric ketogenic diet (EKD) for the following four weeks and this diet consisted of: <20g of carbohydrates per day, the same protein intake as in the first week, while most of the calories were coming from fat. Their VO2max remained unchanged when comparing week 1 of EBD with week 3 of EKD. Their respiratory coefficient dropped from 0.83 to 0.72 from EBD week 1 to EKD week 4.

The athletes managed to drop glucose oxidation three fold (15.1 mg/kg/min to 5.1 mg/kg/min from EBD-1 to EKD-4. This means that they used three times less glucose to create energy). The muscle glycogen (glucose storage) usage went down four-fold. This means that they used four times less glucose from their muscles for energy needs. Their aerobic endurance exercise was not compromised after being 4 weeks in ketosis.

Table 1. Maximal Oxygen Uptake ($\dot{V}o_2$max) and Endurance of Trained Subjects after Eucaloric Balanced (EBD) or Ketogenic (EKD) Diets

	$\dot{V}o_2$max				Endurance					
	$\dot{V}o_2$ L/min*		RQ†		Duration (min)		RQ		$\dot{V}o_2$ (L/min)	
Subject	EBD-1‡	EKD-3	EBD-1	EKD-3	EBD-1*	EKD-4	EBD-1	EKD-4	EBD-1	EKD-4
Mean ± SEM	5.10 ± 0.18	5.00 ± 0.20	1.04 ± 0.02	0.90 ± 0.02	147 ± 13	151 ± 25	0.83 ± 0.01	0.72 ± 0.02	3.18 ± 0.19	3.21 ± 0.18

*$\dot{V}o_2$ = mean oxygen uptake per minute from 30 minutes to exhaustion.
†RQ = respiratory quotient, mean from 30 minutes to exhaustion.
‡EBD-1 = within three days of admission for $\dot{V}o_2$max, end of first week of eucaloric balanced diet for Endurance; EKD-3,4 = after three and four weeks of eucaloric ketogenic diet, respectively.

The researchers conclude that the athletes' adaptation to a ketogenic diet led to an increased conservation of carbohydrates stores (both as glucose and muscle glycogen) and made fat the primary muscle substrate during exercise.

Volek [96] provides support for the research of Phinney [97] conducted a few decades ago. The graph below was created by Jeff Volek based on the data he got from other studies. It basically followed 300 individuals including elite athletes to determine their peak fat oxidation per minute. To better understand this, think of a normal athlete during a marathon. One of the points on the graph (see below) is the maximum amount of fat that an athlete can oxidize (burn) every minute during competition, correlated with oxygen consumption (ml/kg/min).

As you can see most of the subjects in the study were able to burn 0.4 - 0.8 grams of fat per minute. Okay, let's think in terms of marathons again. Say that a normal athlete will burn 0.8 grams of fat per minute and that he will finish the marathon in 4 hours. 4 hours is 240 minutes. This means that the athlete will be able to burn a maximum of only 192g (0.8*240) of fat during the entire marathon.

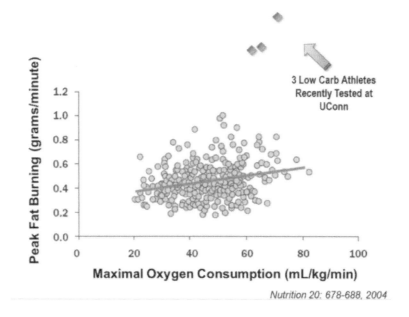

Nutrition 20: 678-688, 2004

Even though there may be high-carb burners who can go up with this amount (and oxidize 1g of fat/min), 190-200g of fat being oxidized for such a long lasting competition is astonishingly low, if you ask me.

Take another look at the graph. See the three points outside the graph? Those are three athletes tested by Jeff Volek. The uniqueness of these athletes is that they are keto-adapted. Their peak fat oxidation rates are 1.5 - 1.8 grams of fat per minute. So, during the same marathon they would burn a maximum of ~430g of fat. They literally burn a pound of fat per marathon. Again, it is quite a difference.

Think of it this way. Keto-adapted persons will burn fat for energy most of the time, either the fat from foods ingested or from body fat. If a fat adapted person requires 2,500kcals to make it through the day and if 90% of that energy is from fat sources, this means that the person would burn ~2,250kcals from fat. That is 250g of fat per day (given that a gram of fat yields 9 kcals).

Under these conditions, a keto-adapted person would be able to burn 250g of fat per day with moderate exercising (no-marathons included). So, a keto-adapted person could burn more fat per day than a high-carb marathoner would do during a competition. This is just to put things in perspective.

If the calories are restricted and if the fat does not come from food, your body will have to shunt it from its own fat storage to get the energy it needs. And it will do so pleasantly.

Peter Attia [2] says that he's doing most of his long-hour bike runs under fasted conditions carrying nothing but some salted peanuts and/or some branch-chained-amino-acids to make up for the possible loss of muscle tissue (due to the long-term endurance training). He's using salted peanuts to make up for the sodium loss through sweat and/or urine. You can check his presentation to better understand the way he's been training.

Another good source of information for very-low-carbohydrate ultra endurance training and exercising is the website of Ben Greenfield. You should check his experiment in which he completed an Ironman competition under ketogenic nutrition [95]. He's been also working with Jeff Volek in his laboratory in the Department of Kinesiology from the University of Connecticut.

I would recommend listening to one of Ben's podcasts with Barry Murray, which is entitled *The Ultimate Guide to Combining Fasting and Exercise: Everything you need to Know.* You can find it here [99]. In this podcast Barry explains how much it takes for athletes and also for the average individual to become fat adapted (he says that the full process can even go beyond the 1 year mark). Again, how many athletes would go this far?

Barry explains that as one becomes keto-adapted, the human body will start building more mitochondria to support the beta-oxidation processes. I know that this is true because I found research on the subject. For example, this study [100] starts on the premise that high-fat diets induce mitochondrial fatty acid oxidation enzyme in the muscle. The researchers wanted to see the effects that higher free fatty acids have on muscle mitochondrial biogenesis.

They observed that feeding mice with high-fat diets plus injecting heparin to increase the free fatty acids leads to higher mitochondrial biogenesis in the muscle.

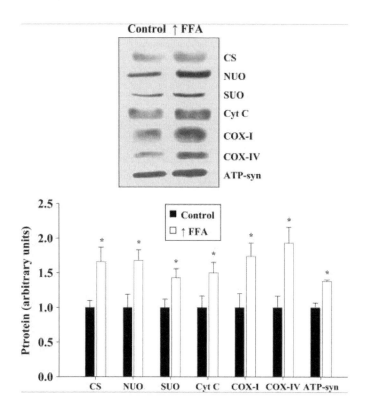

Basically, the image above [100] tells us that there is an increased expression of various enzymes in the mitochondria as a response to higher plasma free fatty acid levels. This may not be the best representative study because it was conducted on mice and because of the methods the researchers used to increase the free fatty acid levels in the plasma of the mice, but it is a good start into researching this subject.

There is another study from 2006 [101] which shows how hypocaloric ketogenic diets enhance brain metabolism and increase mitochondrial biogenesis. Again, the study was conducted on mice. Other studies done on mice [102] [103] [104] reveal the same increased biogenesis of mitochondria under ketogenic diets.

The bottom line for higher performance with high-fat-very-low-carbohydrate nutrition is that athletes need to allow the body to become keto-adapted, thus create all enzymes necessary and possibly increase mitochondrial biogenesis to support the fat burning metabolism. This process could take somewhere from a couple of weeks to a couple of months (and even 1-2 years). This is highly dependant on the current level of physical fitness of the athlete, as per Barry Murray [99].

I would like to further address the issue of strength training under ketogenic nutrition. I will now talk about strength training from the nutritional perspective. I will address it from the exercise perspective in the next section.

Nutrition and Performance for the Keto-adapted Strength Trainee

The common belief is that someone who wants to increase muscle mass has to spend huge amounts of time in the gym and has to increase protein intake as well as carbohydrate intake. This is why there are so many protein shakes and products that are both rich in carbohydrates and in protein. Many of the "gainers" who increase bodyweight in a relatively shorter period of time are basically gaining fat and some muscle, usually very little, if at all.

The next thing our body-builders do is that they have a cutback period after the gaining period, where they lose fat and try to preserve the smaller muscle gained. The ketogenic diet is usually used by the muscle building community in the cutback period because the gainers know that they will lose fat adopting this type of nutritional approach.

I find it not normal to gain 10 pounds of body weight, little of which is muscle and then try to lose most of it and keep only the muscle. Is this rational? Besides, the metabolic stress for this gain/lose "thing" is quite substantial and the long-term effects may not be positive.

It is quite easy to gain weight with the high-carb-high-protein products because we know that the fat storage mechanism (lipogenesis) is not very energy demanding. Besides, the maintenance of the fat storage (adipose tissue) is not energy demanding.

Another reason (my reason) for this gaining approach is that these individuals would not be able to motivate themselves while trying to gain only lean tissue. This process, if done correctly and naturally, is long-lasting and the results are not easily visible. Muscle building is a very slow process and humans like to achieve results the easy way.

The literature has shown that ketogenic diets have muscle sparing effects [113]. This means that one does not need increased protein intake just for the sole purpose of preserving muscle tissue. Phinney and Volek [5] recommend between 1 to 1.5 grams of protein intake per kilogram of bodyweight. So, for example if I weight 70kgs I could consume 70 grams of protein per day, just to maintain my muscle tissues.

If my purpose would be to increase muscle mass I would slightly increase that to 1.5 grams of protein per kilogram of bodyweight. This means that I would consume 105 grams of protein for that purpose. However, if higher muscle mass were only a matter of protein intake, I guess many of us would easily look like the Incredible Hulk because it's easy to eat. We'll later learn that besides nutrition, one important component is exercising. Another requirement is to have good hormonal output. The same importance should be given to the resting period between workouts.

It is also believed that strength training is not possible under ketogenic diets because of the lower glucose levels, which means there would be lower levels of readily available energy for explosive workouts. Let's debunk this myth by taking a little lesson of biochemistry. We'll focus on energy systems and metabolic pathways.

There are three energy systems that we use when we exercise: the ATP-CP system, the anaerobic system, and the aerobic system. The purpose of the three energy systems is to provide ATP through metabolic reactions which are done in the presence or in the absence of oxygen.

The first two systems, the ATP-CP and the anaerobic system (anaerobic glycolysis), work in the absence of oxygen. The difference between these first two is that the ATP-CP system does not output waste products, while the anaerobic system will produce lactic acid as a waste product.

On the other hand, the aerobic system needs oxygen and its waste products are carbon dioxide and water. Here's a simple graph that shows you the duration of each of these energy systems [105].

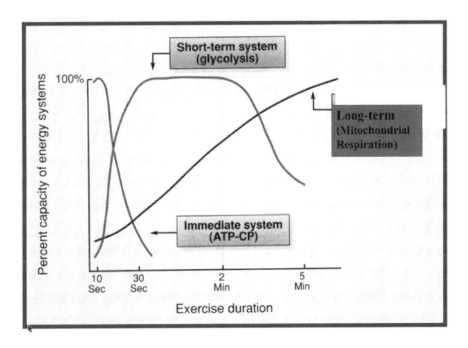

The ATP-CP system uses readily available muscle phosphocreatine (creatine phosphate) to generate energy (re-generate ATP). However, this system of energy is only available for a matter of seconds (10 seconds usually, but some say that it can go up to 30 seconds at most [2]). This is the explosive energy that would make you jump-off out of your skin when a car is about to hit you.

You are using this type of energy system the first few seconds when you are lifting very heavy weights, when you're sprinting, and when you are doing other types of explosive exercises that require the release of a big amount of energy (ATP) very quickly. It's the kind of energy system that ignites you. Once the creatine phosphate storage has been depleted from the muscle (after a few seconds), you shift to the next energy system as you continue to exercise.

The second energy system is the anaerobic system and its purpose is to use glucose through glycolysis (anaerobic glycolysis). The basic idea behind the anaerobic energy system is that it needs to provide energy very fast, faster than your metabolism can use oxygen to power the aerobic system. This type of energy system usually lasts for 2-3 minutes (depending on the athlete's physical condition) and it is required in high-intensity training exercises.

You are using anaerobic glycolysis when sprinting, when swimming, when cycling, and also in other types of high-intensity training. The body is converting glucose to pyruvate and if oxygen is not present, then lactic acid starts to build up.

As it accumulates, this lactic acid is a "non-desirable" product to your body (even though it can be used directly for energy production by the heart muscle and by other organs) and it is taken via the blood stream to the liver. If you exercise very intensively and you build so much lactic acid that cannot be cleaved from the blood stream, your body will try to remove it through vomiting (a good example is a sprinter who runs at 100+% VO2Max or a boxer who punches like crazy).

Okay, so lactic acid has to get back to the liver and be reconverted to pyruvate which will then be converted to glucose through the process of gluconeogenesis. As glucose is created in the liver, it can be taken via the bloodstream back to the muscle cells and the whole process can take place again. This is called the Cori-Cycle (image courtesy of [106]).

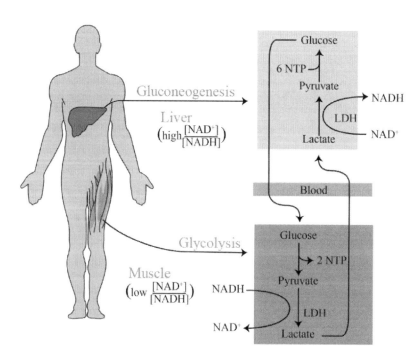

So, these first two energy systems are the most important for our health, if you ask me. I also believe that the aerobic system is not important for building muscle and increasing strength, but it can be important for other purposes.

The aerobic system basically takes glucose or fatty acids and converts them to Acetyl-CoA (remember that I've told you about those?) which then initiates the Krebs Cycle (Citric Acid Cycle) and the ETC (Electron Transport Chain) where it undergoes oxidative phosphorylation to create ATPs (energy). Let's see a quick review of these three energy systems (thanks Peter Attia [2]):

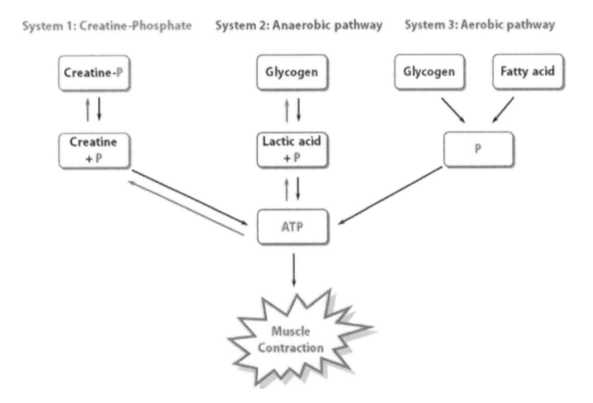

If I didn't lose up to this point, you now have a better understanding of exercising compared to more than 90% of the folks. Okay. Now, let me tell you a story about muscle fibers and how they fit into these energy systems.

Once upon a time there were three types of muscle fibers: type I, type II A, and type II B. The type I fibers are the slow twitching muscle fibers while the type II fibers are the fast twitching fibers. A further classification would put type I fibers as the slow twitching, type II A fibers as the intermediate-fast twitching, and type II B as the fast twitching fibers.

The slow twitching muscle fibers (type I - slow oxidative) are used in aerobic training, in the presence of oxygen to generate ATP for the purpose of fueling steady long-term training, such as marathons and long-bike runs. They are called slow-twitching because they fire more slowly compared to the fast twitching fibers.

The fast twitching muscle fibers (type II) are used in anaerobic training. These types of fibers are used in high-intensity training as they need to provide quick energy in the absence of oxygen. Even though they produce the same amount of energy as the slow twitching fibers [108], they fire more rapidly, which is why the release of a greater amount of energy.

Furthermore, type II A muscle fibers which are the intermediate fast twitching fibers (fast oxidative) can be used for both types of activities: aerobic and anaerobic, while type II B can only be used in anaerobic activities.

Type II B (fast glycolytic) are the fiber types we would like to mostly focus on because they are used along in the ATP-CP system and in the anaerobic glycolysis system, while the other two are used mostly in the aerobic system.

If you want to build muscle, you would have to use your type II B fibers and the only way to do that is to exercise in the first two energy systems. Activities and exercises that exceed the 2 minute mark are aerobic activities and their purpose is to exercise the slow twitching muscle fiber to increase your muscle endurance, and not strength.

Remember the story about the guys who spend many hours in the gym. Most of them are doing aerobics due to the long sets and light weight they use in their workouts. That is a very inefficient way to grow muscle.

Your muscle needs to get the minimum effective dose that would trigger an adaptive response (which is activated during resting periods) and will build more muscle. Next time when you train with heavy weights, you'll be more prepared (aka increase the weights).

Any addition to the minimum effective dose is a complete waste of time. There is ton of research on the minimum effective dose and on how people who workout with weights for 12 minutes a week (1 workout) get the same (if not more) results than those who do several longer workouts per week [30].

Let's not get far from the subject as I will come back to this later. So, the most important characteristics of the three types of muscle fibers are (image courtesy of [109]):

Fibre Type	Type I fibres	Type II A fibres	Type II B fibres
Contraction time	Slow	Fast	Very Fast
Size of motor neuron	Small	Large	Very Large
Resistance to fatigue	High	Intermediate	Low
Activity Used for	Aerobic	Long term anaerobic	Short term anaerobic
Force production	Low	High	Very High
Mitochondrial density	High	High	Low
Capillary density	High	Intermediate	Low
Oxidative capacity	High	High	Low
Glycolytic capacity	Low	High	High
Major storage fuel	Triglycerides	CP, Glycogen	CP, Glycogen

For muscle gains we want to workout our fast glycolytic (type II B) muscle fibers. The most important thing that you have to know is that you need to provide a highly intense short lasting muscle stimulus so that you exercise in the first two energy systems (ATP-CP and Anaerobic Glycolysis).

The proponents of high-carbohydrate nutrition say that ketogenic dieters cannot exercise in these first two energy systems because their glucose intake is too low and glucose is needed by these two systems.

But come to look at it from a biochemical perspective, in the ATP-CP system you do not need glucose as it uses ATP and creatine phosphate which are available in your muscle, while in Anaerobic Glycolysis you certainly need glucose.

However, you do not have to have a full glycogen tank to support this kind of exercise. While on a ketogenic diet you are not deprived of glucose (you have constant lower levels of glucose in your blood stream) and your glycogen tanks are not empty either. These would be enough to support the glucose needed for the 2 minutes of exercise.

Your high fat diet is constantly breaking down triglycerides from your fat storage and the result of this process is: 3 fatty acids and a glycerol molecule. The glycerol molecule is a carbohydrate and can be further used either in anaerobic glycolysis, glucose formation (gluconeogenesis) and glycogen build-up [110] [111] [112].

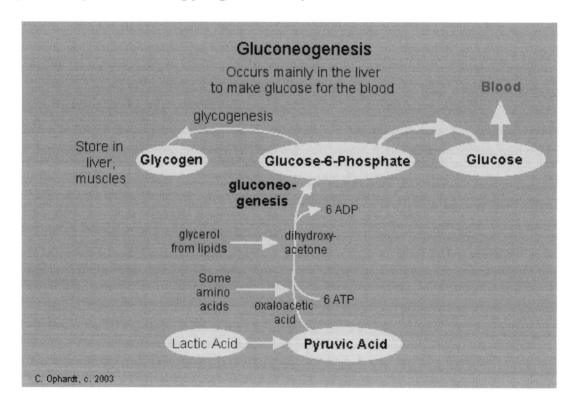

See (above) where the glycerol from lipids (fats) gets converted into DHAP and can further undergo gluconeogenesis and then glycogenesis. The science is always there [111] [112], but the ignorant chooses not to see. High-carb dieters refuse to believe this and will try to find thousands of excuses not to believe it.

As of this writing, there are literally thousands of very low carb athletes and strength trainers. Compare them with the number of high-carb strength trainers and they make up only a small minority. Why? (I propose) because it is not easy to get this mechanism up and running. It is not easy and it takes time to get keto-adapted. It takes time and a lot of applied effort. Few are willing to do it.

I personally did not experience any problems with my sprinting sessions and my strength training. I experienced a setback of 2-3 weeks when I became ketotic but then it all went away and I was able to keep building my strength performance. Take a look at Doug McGuff [30] and his 20+ years of experience with strength training and very low carbohydrate diets. Take a look at Mark Sisson's Paleo approach.

So you know that being ketotic is not an excuse for not being able to build muscle. You need to workout your fast twitching type II B fibers under a high-intense profile and for shorter periods of time. One of the keys (which will be referred to later) to build muscle is to rest properly. Fast-twitching muscle fibers require much more rest time compared to slow-twitching fibers. Here are some activities and the types of muscle fibers they use (image courtesy [107]):

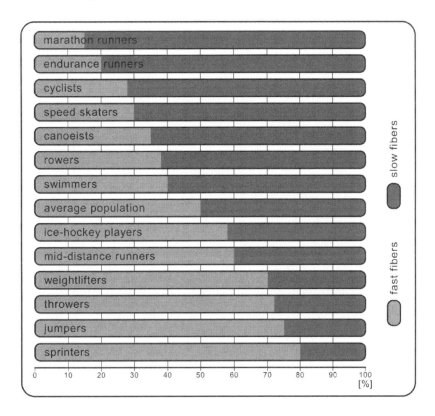

So the bottom categories [107] are the types of activities that you need to do for very short periods of time, such as: weight lifting, throwing, jumping, and sprinting. Similar activities to these will have the same effect. So, be inventive.

There is another myth which says that you are born with a certain number of muscle fibers of each type and those fibers cannot be modified. Up until recently this was a common belief, but it has been proven that strength training can increase the number of fast twitching fibers [30], same as aerobics training can increase the amount of slow-twitching fibers. It is known that gene expression can change as a direct or indirect effect of different factors. This field is called Epigenetics.

Let us review some research to see how the amount of muscle fibers can change as a direct effect of different types of training.

In this study [114], researchers followed 15 male subjects who trained for 4 to 6 weeks, 2-3 days per week on a mechanically braked bicycle ergometer. This was a type of sprint training which consisted of "repeated 30 seconds all-out sprints". This means that the subjects cycled as hard as they could in these sprints which lasted 30 seconds each. They repeated several of these sprints for every session of workout. The resting period between sprints was 15-20 minutes.

Researchers took thigh muscle biopsies before and after the training period. They found that type I fibers decreased from 57% to 48% and type II A fibers increased from 32% to 38%. Researchers also posit that hormonal influences could also be contributing to this change in muscle fibers, besides exercise.

In another study conducted in 1985 [115], the researchers wanted to determine if muscle fiber-type alterations occur when high-intensity intermittent training is used. The subjects were divided into two groups: a group of 24 sedentary subjects (men and women) and a control group of 10 subjects (men and women). The study was done over a period of 15 weeks.

They also tested the subjects on cycle ergometers when doing supramaximal exercise lasting 15 to 90 seconds. They took biopsies from the vastus lateralis (quadriceps) muscle before and after training. The results for the control group remained unchanged. The "exercising" group increased their type I fibers' proportion and decreased their type II B fibers, while type II A fibers remained unchanged.

The researchers also related that the areas of type I fibers and type II B fibers increased for the exercising group. They conclude that high-intensity intermittent training may alter the proportion of muscle fibers and that fiber composition in certain muscles is not solely determined by genetic factors.

There is also this thesis of dissertation from 2010 [116], where P. A. Nader wanted to determine the effects of short-term, high-force resistance training on high-intensity exercise capacity. His study was done on 18 subjects out of which 8 subjects are in the control group and the other 10 are in the resistance training group.

The increase in VO2Max and time to fatigue marginally improved (13%) in the resistance training group. The major drawback of this study is the low number of subjects, but P. A. Nader discusses a lot of literature related to muscle fiber change, which is why I find it a good read.

There is another interesting study conducted by 3 researchers [117] on eight athletes who underwent surgery for knee injuries. The researchers did muscle biopsies before and at various intervals after surgery, while the subjects were recovering. Their type I fibers dropped from 54% to 43%.

There was one athlete who showed a massive reduction in type I fibers (they decreased from 81% at surgery to 58% six weeks later). As he started training he was able to increase his type I fiber count to 85%. I find that pretty amazing. The researchers conclude [117] that it is evident that muscle fiber type composition can change as the type of training and the consistency of training changes.

Two other references [118] and [119] show how skeletal muscle fibers types can increase their count, proportion, and area size as a direct factor of different types of training undergone by the subjects. I believe that further investigation is needed, but one thing is for sure: the genetic package you are born with can be changed. There may be people who are more gifted than other people, meaning that they require less time to grow bigger muscles. But those who have a genetic disadvantage can compensate by working harder. However, the amount of work they have to put-in needs to be more thoroughly analyzed. Yet, there should be no "black and white only" opinions. There are thousands of shades of gray. Anything is possible.

Once again, in order for you to become keto-adapted and experience all the benefits that I've been mentioning throughout this book you have to allow your body the time to become equipped with the proper enzymes and build the mitochondria needed to support such metabolism.

So far we have learned that to increase muscle mass (not only in ketosis) one has to focus his/her workout in the first two energy systems, exercising for shorter periods of time at high-intensity levels.

Remember, you want to build muscle mass and not fat tissue. This takes time, but what do you have to lose? Time will pass anyway, so why not do it? In the next part of this chapter, I will talk about *The Big 5* protocol of training [30] that was created by Doug McGuff more than 20 years ago.

The Big 5 Protocol (+resting) and the Surprise Protocol

This protocol is designed for maximum efficiency. It focuses on 1 workout session that lasts ~12 minutes. It is done once a week and its purpose is to exercise the fast-twitching muscle fiber. It's the protocol that I'm currently following.

Doug McGuff's book [30] gives you the full biochemical and physiological manifesto for why his approach works for most of the people he works with. But let's focus on the workout part. He describes two types of workouts in his book: one with free weights and another one with machines.

There are several protocols that he speaks of, but the most important ones are: The Big Five and The Big Three. I will talk about The Big Five because it is the one that I've been currently following for a couple of weeks.

Since I started going to the gym and lifting weights one year ago, I adopted different approaches. The first 7-8 months I went to the gym 3 times a week, while I was doing kickboxing 2 times a week. So, I was working out at least 5 times a week.

I found that this is way too much for my body to handle, which makes it difficult to progressively increase performance. The Big 5 Protocol is different.

Under the Big 5 [30], you workout your entire body (5 big muscle categories) by doing 1 set to failure, slow movement by using 5 machines or 5 types of free weight training. The 5 exercises are: a cable row, a leg press, a bicep curl, a chest press, and a pull-down exercise.

Here's, for example, the 5 exercises that I'm doing and the order in which I do them:

1. Bicep Curl - 1 set to failure - heavy weights

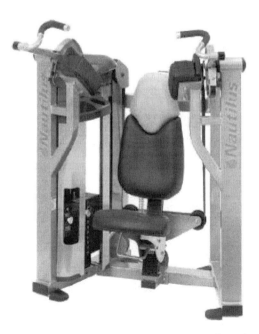

Nautilus Biceps Curl Machine [120]

I start with this machine [120], which is a Nautilus Bicep Curl Machine, and I do 5-6 repetitions with 35kgs (85 pounds) of load. The cadence is 5-8 seconds going up and 5-8 seconds going down. The time under load is critical.

I remember that 1 year ago when I started lifting weights I was doing bicep curls with free weights having a load of 8-10kg (20-25 pounds) on each hand. Something like this [121]:

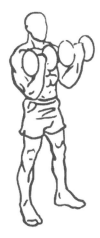

Biceps Curl - free weights [121]

I've changed my approach various times throughout the past 1.5 years. However, I was always following similar patterns. When I started going to the gym I knew nothing and I began training chaotically on all machines. I was exhausting my muscles.

It didn't take long until I revised my thinking and began doing the full body workouts that I mentioned previously, along with adjusting the cadence of the repetitions.

Again, keep in mind four things: heavy weights, shorter periods of time, high-intensity, and a cadence of at least 5/5 (5 seconds up 5 seconds down). This way you train your fast-twitching muscle fibers.

So, to summarize: 1 set to failure on the Nautilus Bicep Curl and then move to the next machine.

I like to do my workouts in a certain order: one pull exercise, one push exercise, one pull, one push, and one pull. This means that there is a pull exercise like the bicep curl, then there is the push exercise like the chest press, then there is the pull exercise like the cable row, then there is the push exercise like the leg press, and the last one is a pull exercise like the pull-down exercise.

You can combine these the way you want and you can choose free weights or machines. It's your choice here, but I would personally choose the machines because of the very low risk of getting hurt.

Before moving on to the next type of exercise, I would like to emphasize that doing this type of workout with a cadence of at least 5/5 (where your movements are slow) will decrease the acceleration, which will lead to a more efficient workout. Think about it (in basic physics terms):

Force = mass x acceleration

Decreasing the acceleration when lifting a heavy weight will make the mass of the load become more difficult to move. This will increase the efficiency of the workout. That is why the cadence has to be at least 5/5 (i.e. 5 seconds for both parts of the repetition). For example on the bicep curl, I lift it for 7-8 seconds, then slowly let the weight back down for another 7-8 seconds.

Experts call this the positive side (when I pull the weight) and the negative side (when I let the weight down). Both of them are important and there are some people who train on only one of them. There are also folks who do the positive, then hold the weight for a few seconds and then move to the negative part of the repetition. There are many approaches to good muscle conditioning, yet many people who go to the gym know nothing about them. For best practices: do your own research.

2. Chest Press Machine - 1 set to failure - heavy weights

I usually do the chest press as my second exercise. If you cannot find a chest press machine in your gym, then you can do the bench-press exercise with free weights, but make sure you have a spotter to help you in case it becomes difficult.

Regardless of the type of exercise:

How do I know how much weight to start with?

Use the 1 rep-max (1RM) assessment. 1RM is basically the max weight-load with which you can do 1 repetition. For example, my 1RM for the bicep curl is 40kgs on the Nautilus Bicep Curl Machine. Once I know this, I will do my 1 set to failure with 80% of that weight as slow as I can.

So, I should do my bicep curl set with 80% of 40kg which is 32kg. However, I do it with 35kg and it is quite difficult, but it maximizes efficiency.

Once you know your 1RM do your 1-set to failure/exercise with 80% of the 1RM.

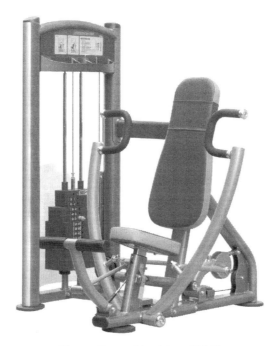

Chest Press-Machine [122]

This is an example of a chest press machine [122]. There are variations of this product and they will all achieve basically the same result. The same idea is to be followed: load the machine with 80% of your 1RM and do 1 set to failure with a 5/5 cadence or more (a.k.a., very slow movements). This is how you focus on working-out your fast-twitching muscle fibers. In case you do not have access to this type of machine, you can always use free weights. Again, be careful [123].

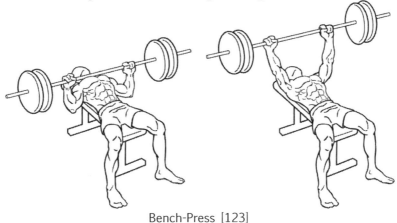

Bench-Press [123]

3. Pull-down (either wide or close grip) - 1 set to failure - heavy weights

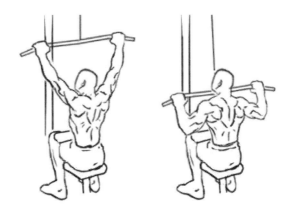

(Wide Grip Pull-Down [124])

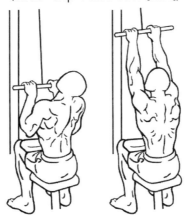

(Close Grip Pull-Down [124])

I believe the images are self explanatory [124]. A good alternative for the pull-down machine would be doing very slow pull-ups/chin-ups [125] (with your body weight or with extra added weights) and/or barbell bent-over [126].

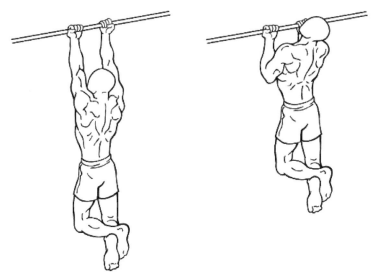

Chin-ups/Pull-Ups [125]

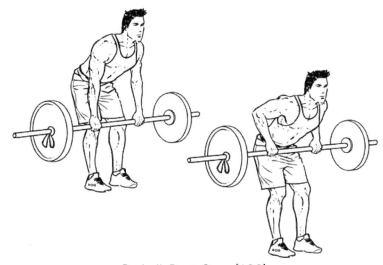

Barbell Bent-Over [126]

4. Leg Press Machine - 1 set to failure - heavy weights

The fourth exercise from the Big Five Protocol is a push exercise, the Leg Press [127]. I now do this exercise with a load of 200kg which is approximately ~440 pounds. A good free-weight alternative for the leg-press machine is the squat [129] (some folks believe it is superior to the leg-press machine).

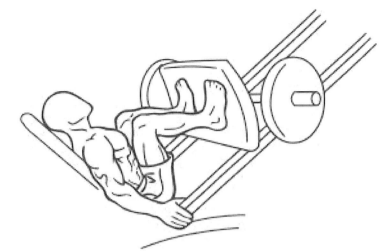

Leg Press Machine [127]

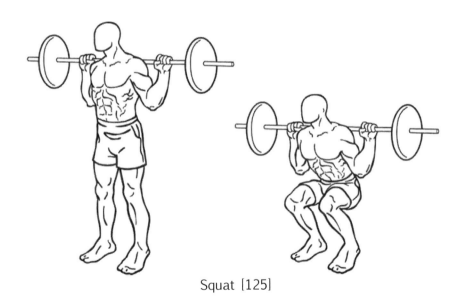

Squat [125]

5. Seated Cable-Row - 1 set to failure - heavy weights

The last exercise of the Big-Five protocol of Doug McGuff [30] is the seated cable row exercise [126]. Two good free weight alternatives to the seated cable row can be the barbell bent-over (see above) or the dumbbell row (either one or two arms - see below).

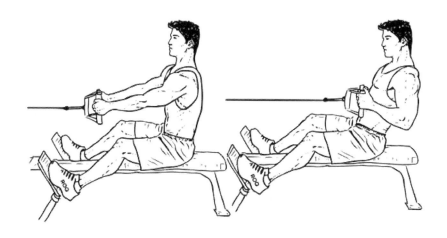

Seated Cable-Row [126]

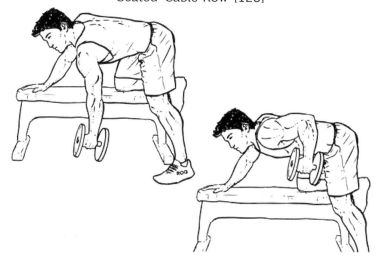

Dumbbell Row [126]

This is, basically, The Big Five Protocol [30] that I'm currently implementing for my strength training practices. This type of training will not be effective and will not lead to the best results if proper rest is not followed.

Doug McGuff [30] keeps emphasizing on the fact that the fast twitching muscle fiber needs far more time to recover compared to the slow twitching one. The slow twitching fiber can recover quickly (minutes to hours), but the fast twitching fiber needs days and sometimes even weeks to recover.

In one experiment conducted by McGuff [30] on one of his clients, he saw an impaired ability of strength training after the subject had rested for 30+ days between training sessions. If that is true, It is amazing and I believe it is something far beyond everyone is doing in the gym.

In most of his works, McGuff suggests that when following his Big Five protocol one should rest for 5 to 7 days between workouts. That is just 1 workout per week! As I was searching on Youtube for different people adopting high-intensity strength training, I found this one [128] where Mike Mentzer shoots a how-to video inside the gym with one of his trainees.

At minute 8, Mike mentions that the last workout of his trainee was 6 days ago and that the purpose of every workout is to increase his strength, which is why he's putting on more weight (as load) for each particular session. I find it very interesting. There have been others who have promoted this type of strength training throughout recent history.

Mike Mentzer's sessions were longer than the Big Five and it encompassed more types of exercises for various muscle groups. However, the similarity between his type of training and Doug's is that they use heavy weights, they do sets to failure, they maintain a cadence of at least 5/5 (5 seconds up and 5 seconds down), and they also use longer resting periods.

Doug McGuff [30] also says that you will know when you're ready to go back to the gym for another session because you'll feel it. I know this may sound a bit "esoteric" but I've personally noticed it in my training. A few months ago when I was hitting the gym 2-3 times a week doing this type of strength training I felt quite fatigued, I felt that I was never fully recovered, which is why I was not able to efficiently increase the load with every session.

Now that I do 1 or 2 workouts per week (sometimes) and I only do the Big Five, I feel quite motivated and prepared after 5-6 days of rest. And I can also increase the load quicker, from one week to another. One of the key ideas behind this type of training is that all the magic happens in the resting period.

When you provide the stimulus during your workout (heavy load, shorter period of time, and intense workout) this will trigger an adaptive response that will manifest itself during the resting period. The adaptive response will consist of your brain releasing signals to your body so that testosterone, growth hormone, IGF-1 and other important hormones are produced at a higher rate with the ultimate purpose of building muscle.

While you are at rest, your body builds up muscle so that you are better prepared when going to the gym next time. Let's see some research on strength training and its effects on testosterone production as well as other hormonal changes. Most of the research that I've found says that there is a positive correlation between strength training and testosterone levels.

In this study [129] nine elite weight lifters were followed for two years to determine their neuromuscular and hormonal adaptations to prolonged strength-training. Researchers have seen increases in the circulating levels of serum testosterone, luteinizing hormone, FSH, and testosterone to serum SHBG. They concluded that prolonged intensive strength straining may influence the pituitary and hypothalamic levels which leads to higher serum testosterone levels.

Another study [130] wanted to test how serum growth hormone (GH) and testosterone (T) respond to progressive resistance strength training programs. They measured basal levels of GH and T (after 12-h of fasting) in young and elderly adults before and after 12 weeks of training. During each session they worked-out all major muscle groups for 45 to 60 minutes doing 3 sets of lifting with 8-10 repetitions per set. They also measured post exercise serum levels of these markers.

Researchers reported that the basal levels of growth hormone increased by 44.9% in the young and by 3% in the elderly. They've also seen increasing levels of GH before and after exercise. Their basal T levels decreased in both younger and elderly while T levels slightly increased in both groups when compared before/after exercise. They concluded that strength training can induce testosterone and growth hormone released no matter the age, but that elder subjects respond differently from younger subjects.

In this article [131], Dr. Mercola describes various benefits of super slow strength training. He talks about the importance of intensity when exercising, the principles of high-intensity interval training, the recurrence of this type of training (a.k.a. how many times you should do it on a weekly basis), as well as his version of the Big Five. I suggest you read it.

Another recent article from 2014 [132] shows how resistance training has the ability to restore muscle sex steroid hormone steroidogenesis in older men. The researchers followed 6 young subjects and 13 older subjects and they took muscle biopsies from their vastus lateralis (quadriceps) muscle at basal state.

The older subjects did resistance training for 12 weeks. The researchers took muscle biopsies 4-5 days after their last exercise session. When comparing muscular sex steroid hormone levels and steroidgenesis-related enzyme expression, they've noticed lower levels in older subjects at basal rate compared to younger subjects at basal rate.

However, the 12 weeks of resistance training in older men led to significant restoration of hormonal levels and steroidgenesis-related enzymes. The researchers conclude that prolonged resistance training restores the age-related declines in "sex steroidogenic enzyme and muscle sex steroid hormone levels in older men." [132].

These few studies point out that when strength training protocols are followed, they lead to a better hormonal output that further promotes muscle gain.

My point is that if you want to increase muscle mass and force you should do your training in the first two energy systems (ATP-CP and Anaerobic Glycolysis), for shorter periods of time (15-35) minutes, doing full body workouts (The Big Five is an example), using heavy loads (high-intensity), and allowing proper rest between sessions (at least 5 to 7 days).

The next protocol in this equation of muscle gain/fat loss is the surprise protocol. I've been using this protocol for approximately a year and a half, but I've been using it more correctly and frequently in the past two months (ever since I've learned more about it).

The person who inspired me to focus on this protocol is Dr. Jack Kruse, a prestigious neurosurgeon from the United States. His protocol is Cold Thermogenesis.

CT refers to exposing your body to cold in different ways [133]. You can either do it using ice baths (where you put ice in the cold water of your bath tub, you can do it by taking very cold showers (I do cold showers for 5-10 minutes twice a day), by doing long runs barely naked (I'd recommend protecting the extremities of your body in this case) and you can also do this by drinking very cold water.

Now, I have to take no responsibility for you doing this. I do not encourage you to do it without the approval (consent) of your physician and I would recommend doing a lot of research (as I did) before jumping into it.

So basically CT is exposure to cold. According to Dr. Kruse [131], when you do this, your body starts burning more fat and releases more energy as heat while ATP production is decreased. I would deeply encourage you to read Jack Kruse's *Cold Thermogenesis* [131] protocol to better understand the bio-chemistry and our body's reaction to cold exposure. It is amazing.

It basically triggers a cascade of hormonal releases which starts in your brain and goes throughout your body. This pathway is also tied to the mechanisms of leptin as it has a very big influence on it. Through cold exposure one is able to recover leptin sensitivity and eventually cure diabetes and obesity, as Dr. Jack Kruse explains. However, to work efficiently, one would have to use a Paleo approach to nutrition and high-intensity strength (resistance) training.

I personally did all three together: the resistance training, the ketogenic diet, and CT through very cold showers. Even though I increased my fat intake drastically and reduce my carbohydrate intake significantly (less 20g of net carbs per day), I was able to maintain the same bodyfat and slightly increase my muscle mass with 1 workout per week.

A very good and in-depth research of thermogenic mechanisms and their hormonal regulation was done by Silva in 2006. See [134]. Another research study done by the same Enrique Silva discusses thyroid hormone control of thermogenesis and energy balance [135]. It is definitely worth looking into Lowell and Spiegelman research from 2000 [136] where they adopt a molecular view of energy production as ATP and heat and how they are influenced by thermogenesis.

As I was becoming more curios about this protocol, I found out about Wim Hof, who is the perfect example of cold adaptation from our days. This guy broke records after records of cold exposure, from staying immersed in ice for more than an hour, to climbing mount Kilimanjaro in his shorts, to running a full marathon (again) in his shorts above the polar circle in Finland, as well as to engaging in other extreme activities which prove his capacity of long-term cold exposure [137].

Here's a quick shot from his Finland marathon [138]:

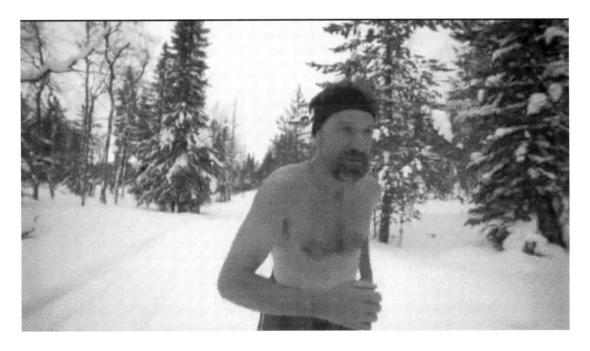

Wim says that cold is his friend. It appears that to be true because researchers from Radboud University Nijmegen Medical Center from The Netherlands have conducted a study on Wim Hof to investigate whether a special concentration technique employed by him can influence the anatomic nervous system activity as well as the innate immune response [139].

They have measured his cytokine response before and after 80 minutes of full body immersion in ice and while Wim practiced his meditation techniques. They have also measured his *in vivo* (live) inflammatory response while in the meditation state and after being administered 2ng/kg LPS (lipopolysaccharides) to see how inflammation levels change in effect to the administration of these bacteria. The researchers compared his results with a historical cohort of 112 subjects who participated in similar endotoxemia experiments (administration of LPS).

They found out that his anti-inflammatory cytokine response was significantly attenuated by his mediation while being immersed in ice. Cytokines are involved in the regulation of the immune system's response to infection and inflammation. Researchers have also observed high cortisol levels during his concentration (which would keep him alert, I assume).

The endotoxemia experiment showed that Wim's catecholamines' concentration (adrenaline, norepinephrine, and dopamine are examples of catecholamines) increased and they were higher compared to any of the 112 subjects in the cohort.

They concluded that Wim's meditation and concentration techniques appear to evoke a controlled stress response which is characterized by the "activation of his sympathetic nervous system and catecholamine/cortisol release which attenuate the innate immune response" [139]. To me Wim Hof shows how remarkable our body is because he is able to hack his sympathetic nervous system's response to cold exposure. The sympathetic nervous system is a region in our brain which 99% of us cannot control on purpose. Examples of people who can get deeper into the brain are the Buddhist monks.

Other people that show tremendous adaptation to cold exposure are the Sherpas. These are the guys that serve as guides for climbers on the Himalayan Mountains. Sherpas can adapt their body for a trip to the top of the world in basically 2-3 days, while the climbers need to stay a couple of weeks at base camp at the bottom of the mountains to adapt for the trip [133].

According to Dr. Jack Kruse, Sherpas (Tibetan people) show unreal resting energy expenditure and resting energy requirements as they need to eat pure lard and butter when climbing the last 2000 feet of the Everest just to maintain weight. Jack however doesn't mention how much fat in terms of calories they consume.

The key take away on cold thermogenesis is that this ancient pathway, as Dr. Kruse likes to mention it, is extremely beneficial in regaining leptin sensitivity, insulin sensitivity, lowering oxidative stress, burning more energy, burning more fat, and increasing the efficiency of the immune system.

I want to end this chapter by talking about my personal experiment with cold thermogenesis. I began taking cold showers in the winter of 2012 to 2013. I started it mildly and continued progressing from moderate cold to the coldest water possible coming from the tap system (it gets extremely cold in winter and moderately cold in summer).

I became fanatic about these cold showers after reading on Jack Kruse's website. So, about two months ago I started taking cold showers twice a day, once in the morning and the other one in the evening, 1 hour prior to bed. The one in the morning was extreme. I started by brushing my teeth for ~3 minutes under the "freaking" cold water, and then kept on showering for another 3 to 4 minutes. This generally triggered a response of shivering for the next couple of hours.

Shivering makes the body increase resting energy expenditure (you burn more calories at rest compared to a non-shivering state). Besides, the response to cold also triggers the hormonal response that I mentioned earlier. One thing that I do not like about cold showers is the fact that my hands and feet are cold for hours after being exposed to cold. But in the evening it does not matter because I go to sleep after taking the shower.

If you look back at the beginning of this book (see page 8), you can see my DXA scan from Dec. 12, 2013. I did another DXA scan and some blood work on April 1, 2014, and it's not a joke. Before revealing it here, I want to give you some brief facts.

Remember that I said that in January I was in Thailand. My stay there was filled with tons of fat coming from coconut (barbecue coconut especially) and pork. I ate little to no carbohydrates and I exercise very little (some recreational swimming).

Then, from February to April 2014 I increased my saturated fat intake and lowered my carbohydrate intake to less than 20g of net carbohydrates per day. I started eating more coconut oil, butter, dark chocolate, tons of bacon, pork, peanut butter, oil roasted peanuts, and eggs. I lowered my protein intake from the period prior to Dec. 2013. I was eating ~100g of protein per day. My daily caloric intake during this period was 2,500-3,000 kcals according to my food logs.

In terms of exercising, remember that I started following Doug McGuff's protocol The Big Five. This means that I was in the gym once a week (sometimes twice per week). After the Big Five, which lasted about 15-18 minutes for me, I usually did sprinting on the treadmill (high-interval-intensity-training) which lasted 10 minutes. No carbohydrate rich foods were ingested after gym. Also, I did not consume any protein supplements. Just food.

This is how my lipid profile changed from the period Oct-Dec 2013 to the period Jan-Apr 2014. I just want to mention that between Oct-Dec 2013, I ate some vegetable oil which could have something to do with the fact that my LDL cholesterol and my triglycerides were showing the values you are about to see.

Test Name	Value 19.09.13	Value 12.12.13	Value 1.4.14	Unit	Reference
Glucose (serum)	67	71	86	mg/dL	70-115
Total Calcium	9.64	9.15	8.96	mg/dL	8.8 - 10.2
Triglycerides	40	74	106	mg/dL	< 150
Total Cholesterol	162	217	198	mg/dL	< 200
HDL	-*	77.7	84.36	mg/dL	> 35
LDL	-*	124	92.4	mg/dL	< 130
Potassium	-*	-*	4.42	mEq/L	3.5 - 5.3
Magnesium	-*	-*	2.16	mg/dL	1.6 - 2.6
Total Testosterone	-*	-*	463	Ng/dL	72 - 853

-* I was not wise enough to conduct these tests early on. I'm just a bit wiser now.

Okay, now let me give you my subjective (possibly biased) view on this. It appears that my fasting glucose slightly increased. I am not worried about that because it is well within the normal range. I would, however, take some action if I saw it was getting worrisome. Total Calcium decreased from one period to another probably because of the lower intake of dairy products. However, Total Calcium is in the normal range as well.

Total Cholesterol increased in the first period (possibly because of the higher intake of vegetable fats (and oils). This is just an assumption. What I'm mostly astonished by is how my Total Cholesterol decreased throughout December to April while I was significantly increasing the saturated fat intake. HDL-c has improved, LDL-c is significantly lower, and Triglycerides are well within the normal range.

This is totally against the general dogma and the conventional dietary guidelines. Now that I've seen it on myself, I truly believe that higher intake of saturated fat in the context of very low carbohydrate intake and moderate protein intake has a positive effect on the lipid profile.

Also, while I increased the intake of saturated fat and the caloric intake to 2,500 - 3,000 kcals, and taking daily cold showers + exercising once to twice per week for 1 hour in total, my body-fat percentage remained the same and my lean muscle tissue slightly increased.

Below, you can see my DXA scan from April 1, 2014. I would have expected my muscle mass to be lower because of the lower protein intake and because of less exercising. I also thought that my body fat percentage would have been increased. I truly believed that, but it seems it didn't change.

Also, from October to December 2013, I supplemented with creatine nitrate, glutamine, and whey isolate while going to the gym. I wonder what the results would have shown if I'd taken these supplements in the period of January to April 2014.

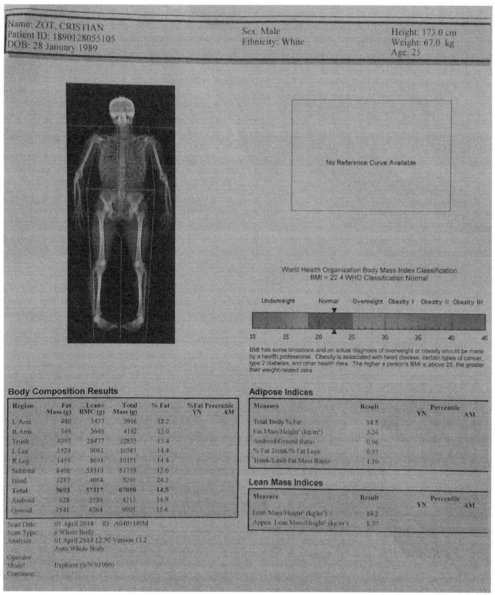

DEXA Scan from April, 2014

My December DXA scan showed a body fat percentage of 14.4%. In April 2014 it was 14.5%. The difference is insignificant in terms of body fat. My lean mass slightly increased with almost two pounds. My next goal is to increase my testosterone levels. I suspect that they were quite a bit lower a few months ago.

In the next chapter I will talk about the types of foods and menus one can eat to sustain the ketogenic lifestyle. Most of the folks know these general menus (like bacon and eggs) so I will focus on the menus and foods that I've experimented with.

Chapter Seven

The Keto Food Chapter

Shopping List - A mess

I'd like to start this chapter in a simple and easy manner. I mean, this is one of the most enjoyable chapters both for me and for you. It's probably the basis of this book and it is the Rx (prescription) for the keto-lifestyle. Let me focus on the psychology of ketogenic diets for a moment.

When I go shopping to the super or hyper market, I find it to be quite challenging. It was even more challenging the first few outings. As you move away from a high-carb diet to a very-low-carb ketogenic diet you also have to move away from the processed food aisles in the supermarket.

My former way of eating (from approximately one year ago, 2013) was somewhat low-carb-ish (e.g. ~150g of carbs per day) 6 days a week and a binging day (when I would indulge in all sorts of carbohydrates). So, purchasing food was not that difficult back then. In my binging days I would frequent the sweet and wheaty aisles. Back in those binging days I was consuming huge amounts of sugar: 10-15 oz. of chocolate, bagels, pizza, french fries, just to name a few.

You'd think it was a very delightful routine. In fact it wasn't because I had to consume a lot of water afterward and the bloating effect which lasted for several hours was very uncomfortable.

As I progressed into keto, it became challenging because, as you know, we are creatures of habit. So, I had to move away from all that sugar to a very limited amount of daily sugar. My initial target in keto was 50g of net carbohydrates per day. This makes shopping a little more challenging!

You have to look for hidden sugars, you have to count fibers, others don't count fibers, you have to know whether or not fibers are included in the "Total Carbohydrates" (it can be different from one country to the next). It takes some getting used to, but it can be done.

Peanut Butter

I remember that I needed to add more fat to my diet, so I added new entries to my shopping list (foods I hadn't consumed before). I started consuming peanut butter. Watch out when you buy these types of butters because some of them can be quite loaded with sugars.

Right now I am in Romania and I eat a type of peanut butter that has approximately 9g of net carbs per 100g (3.5oz). I tried different peanut butters but I got stuck with this one. When you buy your peanut or almond butter, make sure it doesn't have dextrose or other types of added carbohydrates.

If you're really concerned about quality, try making your own peanut/almond/walnut butter. I will give you one of the recipes that I have tried. It's very simple and it takes a ridiculously small amount of time to make.

Dark Chocolate

Another item that appeared on my shopping list was dark chocolate. Since I was used to sweets, I couldn't let them go so easily. I think that dark chocolate is the single most important food that kept me going with this lifestyle. I later found out about its enormous benefits (see what my friend Bill Lagakos writes here [140] and here [141]).

I guess I hit the sweet spot with this one because I got it right from the very beginning. I found the type of chocolate that is decent in the carbohydrate count and it tastes excellent (and it's pretty inexpensive).

Most of my shopping is done at a European supermarket chain called Auchan. It's French-based and it can be found in many countries in Europe. Besides offering products from different manufacturers, they have their own products as well. These products tend to be cheaper because there are no "middle-men" involved.

One of these products is Auchan Chocolat Noir 85%, which is an 85% cocoa dark chocolate and it costs ~$1.5 per 100g. It's very high in fat (52g) and in fiber count (13.2g). They list 16.8g of total carbohydrates. I do not think that you can easily find this product in other places of the world besides Europe. They also make the variant with 72% cocoa and 99% cocoa.

They also have a 76% dark chocolate product with small bites of orange, which is a killer if you ask me. It has 28-30g of carbohydrates per 100g. You could easily eat half of it at once and you'd still be able to maintain <50g or even <30g per day, if you know how.

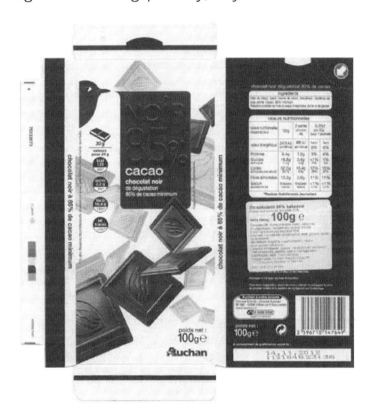

There are other types of dark chocolates that are more easily obtainable. One example would be Weinrich Dark Chocolate. You can look on their website to see the variety of dark chocolates they produce. This is of a higher quality compared to Auchan, but the price is higher as well. I usually get Weinrich Black 85% Cocoa at ~$1.8 per 100g [142].

If you look on Amazon, you can find tons of dark chocolate products, most of which I guess are quite good. Since there is such a large variety of products, you could easily locate the one that fits your needs and tastes. Lindt Excellence or Hershey's products are examples of chocolate that many people prefer. However, they are more expensive than the ones I mentioned above. Later in this chapter, I will also provide the recipe for dark chocolate that I've been experimenting with.

I'd like to remind you to always have the big picture in mind. An example is that 100g of unsweetened cocoa powder should have between 10 - 20g of net carbohydrate, high fiber content of 25 - 35g, and high fat content. If you want to maintain ketosis, make sure you include these values when totaling up your daily macronutrient counts.

Cheese

Before beginning my experiment, I wasn't consuming too much cheese mostly because it was high in fat and I was eating a low-fat/fat-free diet. However, I started adding it to my daily food consumption and now I eat 50-100g of cheese per day. The type of cheese that you should purchase is very low in carbohydrates (<1g per 100g of product) and higher in fat (22-26g of fat). Make sure it does not have too many ingredients on the label (i.e. make sure it is as natural as possible).

Depending on the amount of cheese you consume, you should always make sure that it does not cause constipation. I personally had some negative experiences with cheese and constipation at the beginning of my experiment. I was consuming ~200g of cheese every day and I was doing high-intensity training (sweating a lot). This was a good recipe for constipation.

I found that adding more fiber (from leafy greens and psyllium husk especially) along with drinking plenty of water will eliminate this problem. The bottom line is that cheese is okay as long as you don't eat too much of it and as long as it does not have unwanted chemicals in it.

Peanuts, Almonds, Walnuts, and Brazilian Nuts

I consume these foods regularly. I usually have 100g of oil roasted peanuts. If you buy oil roasted peanuts, make sure the oil that is used is of superior quality: such as olive oil, palm oil, or coconut. I usually eat

100g of oil roasted peanuts and 50g of cheese as soon as I get up. This is my breakfast in the days in which I have breakfast.

Almonds, Walnuts, and Brazilian Nuts are more expensive if you ask me, but they provide greater health benefits. They are rich in Magnesium and Iron and they are high-fat-high-protein products. In my personal experience, I find it very convenient eating them because you need not to cook them; they are readily available. That's why I use them for breakfast, instead of the more common bacon, eggs, and spinach.

Coconut (you name it)

Aaaa....I believe this is the perfect food. There are many coconut products that are recommended not only in high-fat diets but in all diets. There is coconut oil which can be used both internally (eaten) and externally (applied to the skin).

I cook with coconut oil, olive oil, or butter. All of these alternatives are excellent. Coconut oil is superior to other products because of its higher smoking point and because it is has a special metabolic pathway once inside the body. Coconut oil is high in medium chain triglycerides (MCT) which, according to Dr. Mercola [143], go directly into the liver and get converted into ketones, unlike longer chain triglycerides which have to mix with bile to be converted into ketone bodies.

So, MCTs and products high in MCTs provide readily available energy in the form of ketone bodies. As a bonus, these MCTs do not get stored as body fat. There's a remarkable experiment [86], that I mentioned in a previous chapter, conducted by Dr. Mary Newport on her husband who suffered from Alzheimer's disease. It shows how beneficial MCTs are in managing and reducing the effects of this ugly brain disease. Make sure you do not start with a high consumption of coconut oil as it may create stomach discomfort; your body takes some time to adapt using it.

Another great product that I often use is coconut milk. I usually buy coconut cream and mix it with 3 times as much water to get a good consistent coconut milk. I also use the coconut cream for other cooking purposes (dark chocolate, pancakes).

I also buy coconut flakes. I buy the organic type which has 6-8g of net carbohydrate content. I use these flakes when I make pancakes and also when I eat protein bars (I have one bite of protein bar with one teaspoon of coconut flakes).

I sometimes buy whole coconuts, crack them, and eat the meat inside them. These whole coconuts tend to have little water in them because they are aged, and as they are older they will have lower water content. Make sure that before buying them you check that they are not cracked because if they are, they can be spoiled. The cracking process is quite "exhausting" as it can take 10 to 15 minutes to get the meat out of a coconut.

Here's a video [144] where this guy shows us how to "squeeze" the water out of a coconut, the easy way. This is the first step. Then you will take the meat out. I find that if I eat 50g of coconut meat, I can feel full and have no hunger for an entire day. It's the "ultimate convenience food"!

If you find yourself traveling to an exotic location, you might discover the amazing "barbecue coconut" or "BBQ Coconut". I discovered it in my recent trip to Thailand in January 2014.

So what is barbecued coconut?

It is basically young coconut taken from the coconut tree, barbecued and then crack opened. The magic behind barbecue coconut is that its meat is very soft and flavorsome and that it is water full. Back in Thailand, they kept the barbecued coconut in ice so that when served the water from it would be cool and refreshing. Here's a picture of BBQ Coconut:

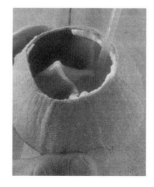

As you can see, the "meat" is easily removable in this one. I usually had 2-3 barbecue coconuts/day. They are fantastic foods. You can usually get them at $1 to $2.5 (30 to 80 baht) depending on the availability.

For example, I was in Phuket, Thailand and the supply of BBQ Coconut was not constant and consistent. There were days with plentiful supply and days when you couldn't find them. The price of them was dependent on the location you happened to be in.

In Thailand you will see merchants who wander along the streets riding their bicycled food stands. They usually sell all sorts of fruits and local products. Some of them will sell you these BBQs for as cheap as $1 (30 baht), while others would ask $2.50 (80 baht) (if you find them in crowded streets). Bear in mind that you should first ask the price of the product and if they ask for 80 baht, politely refuse and offer 50 baht. If they refuse, just go and find another merchant.

When there is good supply of BBQ coconut you will find it almost everywhere, but in the days of short-supply, it is almost impossible to find the product. So, if someone does not want to lower the price, just move along to find another one. Thai people are very willing to negotiate. They are nice people, by the way.

I usually got BBQ coconut for 45-50 baht when the merchant asked 80 baht. When they sell it at 50 baht, I can get it at 30 baht. It depends on my mood and willingness to start a journey along the streets to find the "holy" BBQ.

How do you know it's got a lot of meat inside it?

In my personal experience, I found out that the larger ones have less meat, while the smaller ones have a thicker layer of meat inside them. I'd usually go for the smaller ones because in ~80% of the cases, I was not disappointed with the meat content.

What if you get a bigger one and don't carry a spoon to scrape off the meat from inside it?

They usually give you a straw to drink the cool refreshing water. You can use that straw and push it down the interior of the BBQ Coconut's wall. The straw will accumulate the pasty-fluid coconut meat which you can then suck it up. It's quite simple. You have to be inventive.

If you ever fly to Southern Thailand and land on Phuket International Airport, make sure you look for coconut chips (which are 80 baht). They are delicious and they can be served as on-the-go guilt-free keto food.

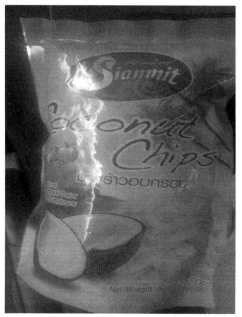

Now you see why I find coconut as being one hell of an amazing food. Besides being high in saturated fats and quite rich in fiber (which is good in high-fat-very-low-carb diets), it's an incredibly versatile food. This statement is not valid for cracking coconuts.

The Everyday Foods

I didn't want to start with the usual meals and foods that are consumed in ketogenic nutrition mostly because it is very common knowledge. Everybody knows about bacon, eggs, butter, pork, and veggies.

I also consume these foods on a daily basis. For example, in some days my second meal (late lunch - early dinner) consists of 3-4 eggs cooked in olive oil or coconut oil with some broccoli cooked in butter and some bacon. The other days I usually have pork cooked in coconut oil or olive oil with broccoli, kale, or leafy green vegetables cooked in butter, and some cheese on the side.

Depending on one's goals for health, nutrition, and lifestyle, these foods can be optimized. For example, if one wants to lose weight, they should restrict calories. However, as I've previously discussed the issue of calories, it's not as important because most of the people who start eating a very-high-fat-very-low-carb diet overeat, but will reduce their caloric intake (in time) as hunger and cravings disappear (partly due to the action of grehlin, LPL, Insulin, and Leptin).

These foods (pork, butter, avocado, eggs, and cheese) are high in saturated fat and they are part of the prescription for the ketogenic diet. You've learned from Phinney and Volek [5] that saturated fat becomes the primary fuel in these diets, so it's safe to consume it. I find these foods as the basics of ketogenic nutrition and the variety in which you can combine them and cook them only depends on your imagination and the time you have for spending in the kitchen.

Meal Plans

People ask me about daily or weekly meal plans when following the ketogenic lifestyle. But there is no meal plan. There are no rules for having "n" number of meals per day with "n" snacks. As Dr. Eric Westman [145] likes to put it:

"Eat whenever you feel hungry, stop when you feel satisfied."

You don't have to eat 3 meals a day; you don't have to snack if you don't want. The most important thing that you have to keep in mind is the carbohydrate content, as I have stated throughout the book. I would not advise for "cheat" days. You do not actually need them.

If you're able to go for a month of strict ketosis, there is a high probability that you stop craving sugary foods. With ketosis you can find a substitute for every high-carb product you can think of.

If you want to eat bread, it can be made from flax seed flour, from almond flour, and from coconut flour, just to name a few. The same thing applies to pizza and pancakes. In terms of sweets, possibilities are limitless. There are a lot of natural sweeteners and tons of websites with guides for ketogenic recipes. Why would I want to re-invent the wheel here?

To re-iterate: I find "re-feeding" (carb loading) days as useless "exercises". You can get all the "satisfaction" you get from binging (cheating) days if you replace those meals with their ketogenic substitutes. And you'll still be in ketosis and not have to suffer from bloating, excessive thirst, and trying to get back into ketosis.

My Daily Meal Plan

The days in which I eat breakfast, I usually want to do it fast and don't want to spend time in the kitchen cooking first thing in the morning. That's why I have:

~100g of oil roasted peanuts (or cashews, or walnuts, or almonds, or the like) and
50-60g of hard cheese.

The peanuts usually have 6-7g of net carbohydrates, while the carb count in cheese is <1g (so it's almost irrelevant). I always have a simple or bulletproof coffee in the morning.

I usually do not have lunch, but when I go to the gym in the afternoon, I sometimes have a post workout snack which consists of a low-carb protein bar with 5-6 teaspoons of dry coconut flakes. I sometimes have a whey isolate protein shake (a recipe that I'll share later). Sometimes I snack on coconut meat (30-40g).

Another snack that I opt for and which I enjoy eating is a simple salad made of:

1 avocado (~2g of net carbs/100g)
50g of unsweetened pot cheese (~4g of net carbs/100g)
half of a squeezed lemon (very low carb content) and
a teaspoon of stevia (sometimes).

Again, I usually have 1-2 meals per day, the first one at 7:30 - 8 A.M. and the other one at 5-6 P.M. And then I have an evening snack.

My second meal, which is at 5-6 P.M. is the "real deal". It's basically:

100-150g of broccoli cooked in butter (or kale or Brussels sprouts, or some leafy greens) (4-7g of net carbs)
150g-200g of fat meat cooked in coconut oil (pork or beef, rarely chicken) (no carbs)
50-60g of hard cheese (<1g of net carbs/100g)
and sometimes 150g of cabbage salad (dressing: olive oil, vinegar, salt, and pepper). (6-7g of net carbs)

On some days I have the meal above, while the other days I replace the meat with eggs and bacon. To illustrate:

100-150g of broccoli cooked in butter (or kale or Brussels sprouts, or some leafy greens) (4-7g of net carbs)
*4 eggs and 50-100g of bacon (eggs have <1g of net carbs/100g)
50-60g of hard cheese (<1g of net carbs/100g)
and sometimes 150g of cabbage salad (dressing: olive oil, vinegar, salt, and pepper). (6-7g of net carbs)

My evening snack consists of:

50g of dark chocolate (8-10g of net carbs)
2-3 teaspoons of peanut butter (2-3g of net carbs)
4-5 Brazilian nuts (2-3g of net carbs)

This is just a brief and approximate overview of my meal plan and it varies widely. I usually aim for 25-50g of net carbs/day. There are days when I don't eat (i.e. I do intermittent fasting) just to give my body a break from food. Intermittent fasting (IF) means that I stop eating from one evening to the next.

I usually finish my intermittent fasting period with an 800-1000kcals meal consisting of some peanuts, some dark chocolate, and some cheese. Additionally, I have a small glass of red dry wine and a few

Brazilian nuts. The best thing about intermittent fasting is that you are not hungry and the time you save by not eating leaves you with plenty of time to do other stuff if you're a very busy person. Now, let's talk about some recipes that I've experimented with.

Personal Experiments

The recipes that I present here represent a very narrow list of what you can eat when following this nutrition plan. I found some very useful websites that can give you specific meal plans for ketogenic nutrition:

Keto Approved [146]
Keto-safe Foods [147]
Ruled.me [148]
Ketodietapp [149]
Keto/low-carb [150]

Another very good 20-page quick start guide on ketogenic nutrition, foods to eat, and foods to avoid is written by Duncan Lewis and can be found in Gary Taubes' book [16] or here [151]. The guide also talks about sweeteners, alcohol, and amounts of carbs to consume, but I will also discuss them later in this chapter.

As I recommend recipes and/or menus for ketogenic nutrition I urge you to "think outside of the box". I mean, you now know the most common foods that you can consume on a ketogenic lifestyle. You also know that you should focus on consuming 30-50g of net carbohydrates per day depending on your lifestyle and day to day routine.

I challenge you to start experimenting on your own with these foods. Try crafting recipes for yourself. The recipes that you are going to read about have been taken from different books and/or websites and have been personalized to my own tastes. The recipes that I fully take credit for are: my avocado salad, my fat bomb, and my keto pancakes with cheese and tomato. The rest of them are tweaks of known recipes. Again I won't reinvent the bacon and eggs or the veggies and fat meat recipes that all of you should know about.

My Bulletproof Coffee

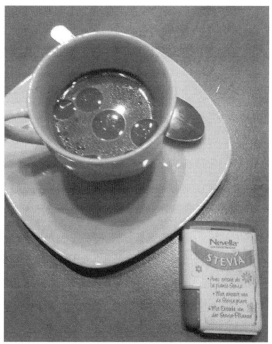
BPC - Bulletproof Coffee

I usually have a normal cup of coffee that is very hot and add 1 stevia pill so it can dissolve quickly. Then I **add 1 tbsp of butter, 1 tbsp of coconut oil and some heavy cream**.

You can also experiment with coconut cream, coconut milk, soy milk, olive oil or any other type of fat that suits your fancy. I encourage you to be inventive. It's far more interesting.

I used soy milk in the days in which I fasted (religiously) and was not allowed to consume animal products.

The basic idea behind this bulletproof coffee is to provide some calories in the form of fat and to suppress hunger. However, hunger suppression is not necessary when you are fat adapted (keto-adapted).

Many keto dieters use bulletproof coffee to skip breakfast and to avoid that feeling of hunger. The average caloric intake for 1 cup of this coffee is highly variable because of the added fat. However, you should know that plain coffee has 0 calories while:

1 tbsp of coconut oil has ~120kcals
1 tbsp of butter has ~100kcals
1 tbsp of heavy cream has ~50kcals
1 tbsp of soy milk has ~8 kcals
1 tbsp of coconut cream has ~50kcals
1 tbsp of olive oil has ~120 kcals

So an average cup of coffee in which you add 1 tbsp of coconut oil, 1 tbsp of butter, and 2 tbsp of heavy cream will yield ~320kcals. You just play in with the values to get your own version of BPC.

My Avocado Salad

My first encounter with avocado was when I started the ketogenic lifestyle. I didn't even know what it looked like and I barely knew of its existence. An average avocado (100g) has:

~150-200kcals
8-9g of total carbohydrate, 6-7g of fiber (thus, 1-2g of net carbohydrate),
~15g of fat, and
~1-2g of protein.

It's almost flavorless and most people consume it in combinations (either salted or sweetened). My avocado salad (sweetened) looks like this:

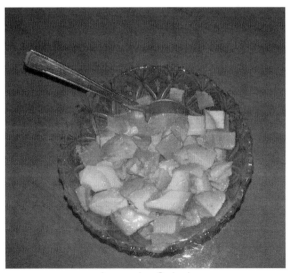
Avocado Salad

What's in it?

1 avocado
1 squeezed lime or lemon juice
1 teaspoon vanilla extract
1 teaspoon stevia (or Erythritol, Xylitol, or other good sweetener).

How do you prepare it?

It's quite simple and it takes less than 5 minutes, as long as you have the ingredients readily available. You just remove the avocado skin and cut it as in the image above. Then you squeeze the lemon or lime, you add the vanilla extract and the stevia. **The caloric content is ~200-250kcals.**

Sometimes I add 50-100g of unsalted, unsweetened pot cheese. It's extremely delicious.

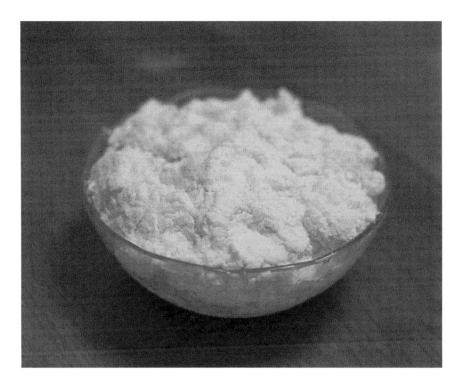

The pot cheese that I use has (per 100g):

~250-270kcals
24g protein

16g fat
3g of carbohydrates

With the extra added pot cheese, the avocado salad has ~450-500kcals.

My Fat Bomb

This is the type of meal where my imagination goes wild. In December 2013 I was 2+ months in ketosis and hadn't experimented with fat bombs yet. Hearing about it and seeing people discuss it on many FB groups and forums made me think of designing my own fat bomb. Here's a "view" of the ingredients:

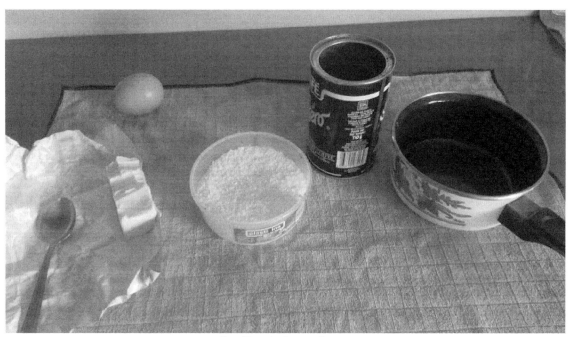

Fat Bomb Ingredients

Here's the list of the ingredients:

30-40g of unsalted butter
30g of coconut flakes
1 tbsp of cocoa powder (unsweetened)
1 egg (you can use 2 if you want)
1-2 tbsp of heavy cream

Cocoa gives a very good flavor to the mix. First let the butter fry in the cooking pan, then add the coconut flakes and mix it quickly. Make sure it does not get burned. If you want you can add a tbsp of coconut oil to make it more fluid. Scramble the egg and add it to the concoction. Make sure that everything is homogenized. Keep mixing until the egg is cooked. Take it from the stove and add the cocoa powder. Mix it until it is homogenized. Add the cream.

For more flavor, you can also use protein powder (I recommend whey isolate because it's very low in carbohydrate count), 1 tbsp of vanilla extract, or 1 tbsp of rum extract. Here's a picture of the finished fat bomb.

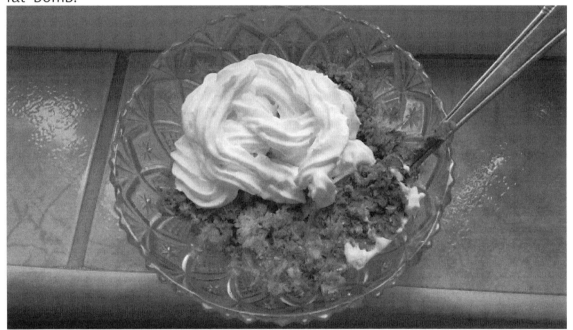
Fat Bomb

Total caloric "damage":

~750-800kcals and ~5g of net carbohydrates. It's quite satisfying and fulfilling.

My Protein Shake

I learned about the fat protein shake from Steve Phinney and Jeff Volek [5] and I added some extra ingredients to the concoction. I find it very delicious. I do not consume it often, but when I do, I usually drink/eat it after a workout (gym or HIIT).

What I use:

1 serving of whey protein isolate (~30g)
1 tbsp olive oil
50g berries
150-200 ml of water (that's like 5-6 oz)

That is the base recipe. However, you can add some coconut milk instead of water. If you use water you can also add 2-3 tbsp of heavy cream.

Here are the basic ingredients:

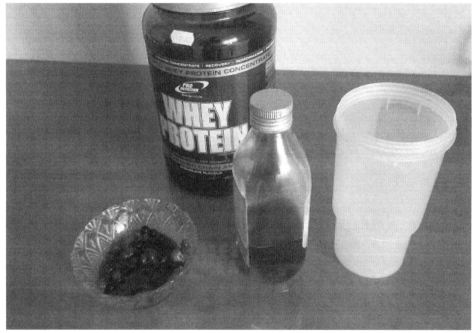
Fat Protein Shake

How do I do it?

I first add 1 serving of protein to the container, and then I add the berries and mix until it is homogenized. Then I add the olive oil and mix it. Lastly I add the water (and sometimes 2-3 tbsp of heavy cream). Here's how the finished product looks like:

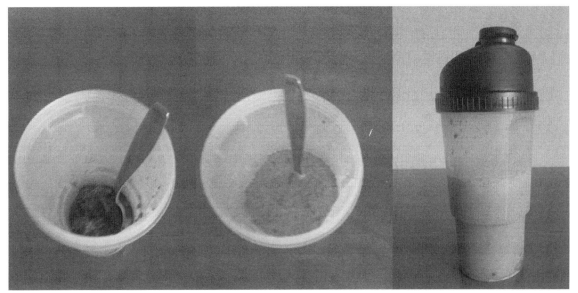

It contains approximately 300-350kcals and 3-5g of net carbohydrate. It has ~23-25g of protein. You can add two servings of protein, but you'll also have to add some extra water. Again, play with the quantities based on your own preferences.

My Keto Pancakes

A couple of days after being in ketosis I realized that I could no longer have those Sundays where I'd basically stuff myself with carbohydrates of all sorts, starting with pizza and finishing up with creamy pancakes with chocolate syrup or peach jam. It was kind of depressing and that made me search for alternative ways to get the flour needed for such types of meals, a type of flour that would satisfy my ketogenic food requirements.

It didn't take me long to discover coconut flour, almond flour, and/or flax-seed flour. So far I've only tried coconut flour. Now, when I make the amazing coconut pancakes, I don't even use coconut flour but coconut flakes. These keto pancakes are amazing, very fat and very delicious.

The first time I made them I wanted them to be very thin. I was used to the thin grain-flour pancakes made by my mother. I didn't get the right recipe from the very beginning so the first experiment was a "flop". I know it's possible to cook them and get thin pancakes, like the ones from wheat flour but, now, I love the thick ones.

The basic ingredients that I use are:

50g of coconut flakes
50-70g of heavy liquid cream
3 eggs

I mix the eggs and the liquid cream and then I add the coconut flakes and mix all of them together. I cook them in olive oil or coconut oil. You can use coconut cream if you do not want to use heavy dairy cream.

You may notice that there is no sweetener here. Yep, it's not needed. Here's how they look. They are basically unsweetened so I can later use them either in a sweet or a salty combination.

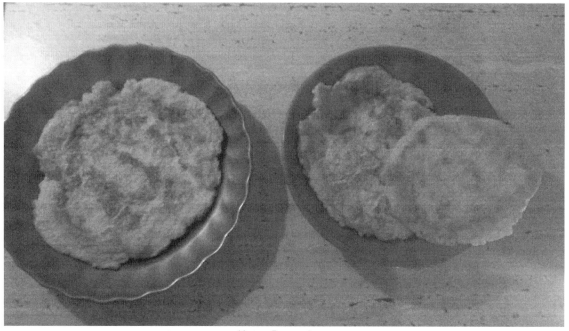
Keto Pancakes

One time I prepared them when I was at my parents' house and my mother joked that they look like just a plain ol' omelet.

There are many recipes over the internet where they add stevia extract, vanilla extract, and/or lemon extract. It depends on how you want to serve them. If you want them sweet then you can add these ingredients mixed with the liquid ingredients. Instead of lemon extract, I'd squeeze a bit of lemon juice just to make them tastier (or one could try using lemon zest).

I prepared the pancakes this way because I wanted to serve them both as salty and sweet. For the salty version, I just added some cottage cheese and unsweetened tomato sauce. Have a look at them below.

For the sweetened version, I just used berries and heavy cream. Looks delicious, right?

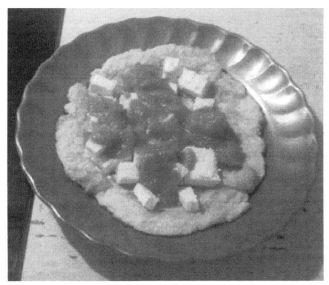
Pancakes - Salty Combo

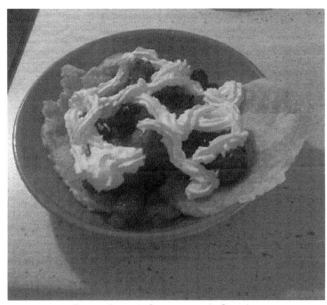
Pancakes - Sweetened Combo

Now, let's look at the calorie and carbohydrate content.

The sweetened combo adds up to ~1000kcals and ~17g of net carbs, most of the calories coming from fat and most of the carbs coming from the berries and the coconut flakes.

The salty combo nets ~1200kcals and ~11g of net carbs, most of the calories coming from fat and most of the carbs coming from the coconut flakes and the tomato sauce.

Here's how my first keto pancakes looked like! At that time I only did the sweetened version of them.

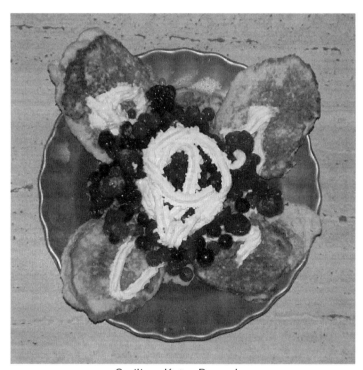

Smiling Keto Pancake

There's this nice video on Youtube showing you how to make gluten free, wheat free coconut pancakes:

https://www.youtube.com/watch?v=gROg24jBJWc

My Primavera Salad (with extra-added fat)

For productivity and time saving reasons I found myself wanting to enhance the FAD chicken salad that I get from the supermarket. We find it here under the name of Primavera Salad (Spring Salad) and it is a combination of chicken breast with salad, cucumbers, olives, tomatoes, peppers, carrots, and cabbage. I would approximate that it has 200kcals and 1 serving is 300-400g of product.

I wanted to add some color to it so I threw in some cheese (100g of cheese) and some bacon/sausages (100g). This is the enhanced version of the Primavera Chicken Salad. The extra-added cheese + bacon does not provide additional carbohydrates, but they add approximately 600-700kcals, three times as much as it had initially. So, the total caloric content is now ~800-900kcals. The carb content comes from the green ingredients, from the tomatoes and from the carrots and I approximate it to be 5-7g of net carbohydrate. Additionally you may add some mayo. Just make sure it is not loaded with carbohydrates. Here's how my enhanced salad looks like.

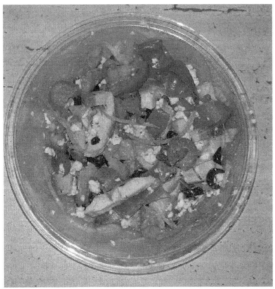

Enhanced Primavera Salad

My Omelet

I guess you all know the bacon and eggs part of the ketogenic lifestyle. Here's what my basic omelet looks like.

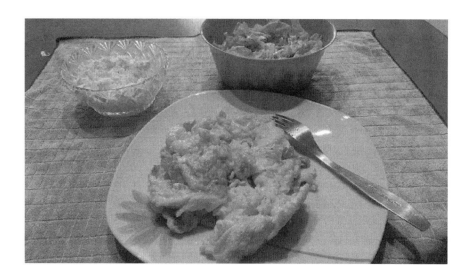

It's usually made of 3-4 eggs and 30-40g of bacon (very fat bacon). I then add some cabbage salad with dressing made of olive oil, salt, pepper, and vinegar and have some pot cheese on the side. Most of the carbs of this meal come from the salad and the pot cheese (100g of pot cheese can have 2-4g of net carbohydrate).

I've mentioned my other main meal that I'm having the other days but I haven't revealed it to you yet. So, here's it is:

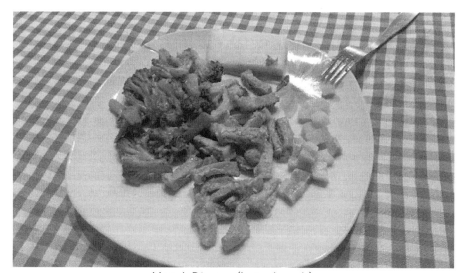

Usual Dinner (Late Lunch)

It's basically 150-200g of pork, 150-200g of broccoli cooked in butter, olive oil or coconut oil, 20-30g very fat bacon, and ~50g of hard cheese. This is a very satisfying high-fat, moderate protein, low carb meal.

Sometimes, after 2-3 days of water fasting, I have this huge load of fat and protein. I basically force myself to eat it. I believe this is where I'm kicked out of ketosis for a few hours, even though not always.

This type of meal is extremely satisfying and I tend not to eat for the following 24 hours mostly because I do not feel hungry. I do not feel hungry when finishing water fasting probably because I take cold showers and probably because I'm decently keto-adapted. It's great not feeling hunger. So, here's the bomb:

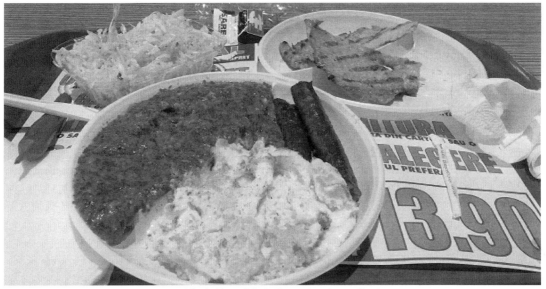

High-Fat, High-Protein, Low-Carb

~200g of spinach (I can't and don't eat all of it)
~200g of cabbage salad (I never it eat entirely)
~150g of grilled chicken breast
~2 eggs made in palm oil
~2 sausages (~150g)

I believe this meal has ~1200kcals as per my rough calculations and the carb content for 200g of spinach+200g of cabbage salad is ~8-12g of carbs. Protein accounts for 60-70g per this type of meal, while fat mostly comes from the eggs and the sausages. Chicken breast is low fat.

Back in Thailand, I had this great omelet for a few times:

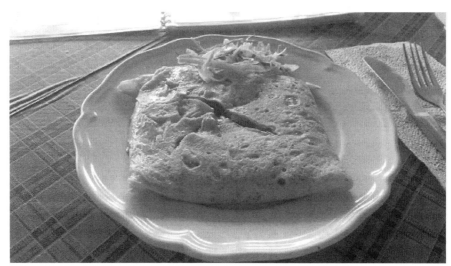

It's made of 3 eggs and it is filled with minced meat, some seasoning, and tomato sauce (unsweetened). It's very satisfying mostly because it is high fat. A rough estimate of macros: ~750-850kcals, 2-3g of net carbs, ~45-55g of protein, and ~55-65g of fat.

My Dark Chocolate

Dark Chocolate is one of my favorite daily treats. As I've told you before, I consume half a bar of dark chocolate 85% cocoa every day. That is roughly ~50g of dark chocolate. The carb content in these commercial dark chocolates is ~15-25g of net carbohydrates per 100g of product.

However, if I make dark chocolate at home, I get very-low-carb-high-fat dark chocolate. Here's what I put in it:

50g of unsweetened cocoa powder (5g of net carbs)
50g of liquid heavy cream (1.5g of net carbs) - you can also use coconut cream
~20g of olive oil or coconut oil
1 teaspoon of stevia (I do not use it always)
10g of dried coconut flakes (~1g of net carbohydrates)

I put the coconut powder in a container and then add the heavy cream. I mix them together for 1-2 minutes. Then I slowly add the olive or coconut oil and mix everything together until they blend. I get this pasty-fatty combination. Then I add the stevia and the coconut flakes.

Sometimes I add 1 teaspoon of vanilla extract and/or rum extract for enhanced flavor.

The last thing to do is to give it shape. I basically take it from the container and wrap it in plastic film. I give it a rough rectangular shape and put it in the refrigerator for 30 minutes to one hour.

I like it a lot because it is intense, it is fat, and it is very low carbohydrate. The net carb count is ~7-8g of net carbohydrates. It has ~400-500kcals. If I eat the entire 130-150g of chocolate I may get "high" (agitated) from the cocoa. It's crazy you know. Here are two versions of my dark chocolate:

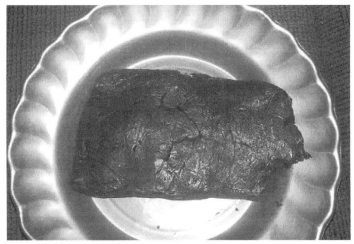
My First Dark Chocolate Experiment

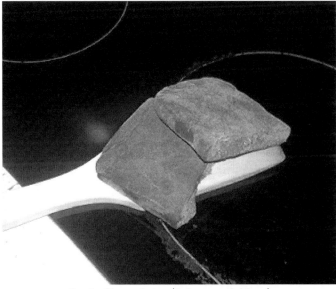
Dark Chocolate (Advanced User)

My Super Simple Almond Butter

Out of frustration that I couldn't find almond butter anywhere in the supermarkets near me, I decided to make my own. I just blended 50g of almonds. I left some bigger pieces of almond unblended so that the end product will be crunchy.

After having the almonds blended, I just added some coconut oil and some olive oil until the whole combination became pasty. Then I added a bit of salt. I wanted a salty product. But if you want to have a sweet product you can simply add some good sweetener like Stevia, Xylitol, or Erythritol, to name a few. And that's it.

I just threw it in the fridge for approximately 1 hour and the surprise was that once I got it out of the fridge it was hard like a rock. Can you guess why?

It is because of the coconut oil. It hardened. It is very crunchy once you get it out of a cold environment, but if you leave it a few minutes at room temperature, it becomes like a butter (hence the name).

Sweeteners

The sweetener that I mostly use is Stevia. It comes in two forms: stevia droplets and stevia powder. I have not had any negative experience so far. Some people say that stevia kicks them out of ketosis. But I do not think this is the root cause of their problem. Maybe some other thing from the diet is doing it. Some other people say that they do not like the taste of stevia.

As far as I know (from the label of my stevia droplets) this product is 300 times sweeter than sugar. 1 stevia droplet accounts for 1 teaspoon of sugar but it basically has 0 carbohydrates. I use 1 droplet for 1 cup of coffee and it is enough to get a decently sweetened coffee.

I use the stevia powder when making dark chocolate, for pancakes, or when I make the sweet version of the avocado salad (avocado, squeezed lemon juice, pot cheese, and some stevia).

There are other alternatives if one does not like or does not want to use stevia. As I've mentioned before you can use [152]:

Erythritol
Xylitol
Mannitol
Sorbitol
Yacon Syrup (I just discovered this one).

You can find them under these names or under different labels. They are very low in carbohydrate content and most of them do not spike blood sugar, but if you really want to know the exact carb content and breakdown, you will have to read the labels for each of the products.

Alcohol Consumption

The most important rule of the ketogenic lifestyle applies to alcohol consumption as well, that is: **go very low carb**.

I surely did not want to practice abstinence while following the ketogenic lifestyle. That is why I wanted to know and to test how exactly alcohol impacts my state of ketosis.

I knew that I had to avoid beer and other high-carb alcohol drinks and that I had to stick mostly with the "pure" alcoholic beverages. After all, men should drink strong stuff if they drink, and not drink beer or high-carb cocktails so that they will go the bathroom all night long.

When you consume alcohol you want minimum impact on your state of ketosis. Good choices are: whisky, vodka, rum, cognac, tequila, red dry wine and any beverage that does not have extra added sugar. Make sure you know or read the label of what you consume. The ones that I mentioned above are the ones that most of the keto warriors prefer.

I do not recommend low carb beers and other un-natural low-carb drinks. If you want some flavor with your strong drink, have some unsweetened lemonade or grape juice.

My experience with alcohol and this lifestyle is to stick to whisky, cognac, red dry wine, and tequila usually along with diet coke. I hate diet coke but, consumed in moderation, I do not believe it causes harm. When I drink red wine, I don't use diet coke.

I also tested the time it takes for my body to be back in ketosis after having alcohol. The results are varying. I usually drink alcohol 3 to 4 hours after a meal and I usually do it at night.

There was one time when I had 150g of whisky and ~50g of diet coke. I tested my urine ketones two hours after the drink and then 4 hours after the drink. My ketone levels were ~1 mmol/L. It's really interesting because I've learned that once you have alcohol, your body puts ketosis on pause for a while and starts focusing on metabolizing the alcohol. Then, it continues with the ketosis.

I've tested alcohol's impact on ketosis and whenever I have small amounts of alcohol, I basically do not get out of ketosis, as long as the drinks are very low carb.

On another occasion I had 300-350g of whisky and 1 diet coke (over a couple of hours). I tested to see if I was in ketosis when I got home and my urine ketones tested negative. After 6-7 hours of sleep, I woke up and checked my ketone levels again. I was back in ketosis.

Basically, every time I drink heavier (300g+ of alcohol), I get back in ketosis the next morning. However, there have only been 2 or 3 of these experiences. There was one night at a wedding (when I had whisky) and another night when I had some tequila shots with a friend. I had l6 or 7 shots (approximately 250g of tequila in total).

Most of the keto dieters that I know unanimously agree that it takes very little alcohol to start feeling the "happiness" effect. That's why I only have 50-100g of whisky or cognac when I have a drink. I also agree on the fact that the dose makes the poison. So be careful when drinking alcohol.

A lot of folks love to hear that wine is a good alcoholic beverage that can be consumed in ketosis. I believe that a glass of good wine is beneficial to health. I personally have a glass of wine every couple of days. The type of wine recommended to stay in ketosis would be dry wine because this tends to have little carbohydrates. My research tells me that dry wine can have 1-4g of carbohydrates per 100g of product. Some types of white wines can be low carb.

The type of wine that I usually have is dry red wine (Cabernet Sauvignon). Drinking one glass of this type of wine, which is approximately 250g and has 7-8g of carbohydrates, I have tested ketone levels immediately after and two hours after drinking it. My ketone levels were unaffected and I was able to stay in ketosis. It showed 3-4mmol/L both immediately after and 2 hours after.

The bottom line is that you can have alcohol and still not affect ketosis and the ketogenic lifestyle. Avoid high-carbohydrate drinks such as liquors, cocktails, beer, etc. Again, the dose makes the poison. So you should keep your alcohol intake (no matter the lifestyle and the diet you have) as low as possible.

You asked, I answered

In this small section of the chapter I will try to address some of the questions that most of you have asked me with respect to this lifestyle. I want to point out that my personal experiences apply to me and that they do not have to be generalized or taken as rules. Here we go.

1. Eating and Drinking Out

I believe that most of the restaurants will provide very low carb options for foods and drinks. You know the foods and the meals you can have. However, make sure that the sauces you are served do not have added sugar. I've personally had some negative experiences when I ordered some Chinese food which consisted of 3 or 4 types of meats soaked in a sauce. The sauce was diabolically sweet so I had to throw it out.

The ketogenic foods you can find in most restaurants are: fat meat (steak, beef, animal organs, etc), eggs, cheese, broccoli, leafy greens, etc.

Don't even try to find low carb pizza or other stuff. You are not likely to find it. You can make these by yourself at home.

There is some Middle Eastern food that I like and it is called shawarma. It usually comes in a bun and it consists of beef or chicken, fries, sauces, and some salads. I always ask for the plate version, without the bun or pita (Libyan bread) and without the fries. So, basically what I get is the meat and the salads. I order some mayo along with it. If you order mayo, make sure you have a degree of certainty of what's in it.

The same strategy applies to hotels. You know the foods you can eat on your ketogenic lifestyle so you can always seek to find them in these menus of the restaurants and hotels you stay while traveling.

2. Eating while Traveling

Whenever I travel, there are some foods that I can always carry with me without having the fear of them getting spoiled. However, since I've not been hungry lately, I only eat with the purpose of not losing weight.

I usually carry some form of nuts, almonds, or peanuts. I like to eat oil roasted peanuts while traveling. I can also have a very low carb protein bar on the go. I've heard people carrying butter in soap boxes and eating them with teaspoons. I know that some people carry bacon with them while traveling. However, make sure the bacon is smoked so it will not spoil quickly.

If you are served food in the plane you can always have the high-fat low-carb items on the menu. While flying for 10 hours to Thailand back in January 2014, we had been given warm meals, coffee and different juices.

I opted for black coffee with some milk. I sweetened it with stevia. I also had tomato juice (unsweetened). The Russian airline was very hospitable to its customers. The warm meal consisted of all sorts of foods out of which I eliminated the bread, the pasta, and the sweet stuff. I was left with butter, eggs, meat, and some veggies.

3. Optimal Macro Levels

These are very important in ketogenic nutrition. The basic of the basic is to eat: at least 60% fat, <10% carb, and the rest of % as protein from the total caloric intake. I usually go for 70% fat, 20-25% protein, and 5-10% carbohydrates. These levels can vary from person to person and can depend on the level of activity and purpose of the diet.

If you workout often, you can sneak some carbs-in right after the workout because they will be used to fill in the glycogen tank and not for storage as fat or to spike insulin levels. However, this is not necessary and you should only do it for your love of eating carby stuff. If you decide to sneak in some carbs, make sure you don't go and eat 200-300g of carbs after 15 minutes of running. You know that's not okay.

Instead, you could have some dark chocolate, a few spoons of peanut butter or a protein bar after a workout. You could also have some berries with fat cream. Make sure you do not exaggerate.

4. What do people do wrong?

There are a lot of folks complaining that it is really difficult for them to get into ketosis, that they feel sick, or that they are not able to maintain this lifestyle.

One of the most common mistakes is that people do not know their macros. It takes a bit of effort to do some math in the beginning so that you know everything what you eat in terms of calories, % of fat, % of carbs, and % of protein. I believe this is necessary in the beginning. After a few days one will easily know everything they eat and counting will no longer be necessary.

Another common mistake relates to sodium intake. With inadequate sodium intake your body does not retain water and when you eat very low carb it can lead to feelings of fatigue, light-headedness, and headaches.

This is easily correctible by adding a few grams of sodium in the form of chicken broth, extra salting of food, or having some tomato sauce with a few grams of salt (which I find to be the most delicious).

Another common mistake is that people do not stay enough into ketosis to start feeling the benefits (ex: no hunger and no cravings).

You do not actually need carb refeeding days. I believe that if you have carb refeeding days every week you are less likely to become keto-adapted and it will be more difficult for you to stay in ketosis, which makes me think of....

5. Ketosis vs. Ketoadaptation

Ketosis is simply the state in which your body's primary source of fuel is derived from fat. Ketoadaptation instead is when your body has stayed enough time in ketosis (without being kicked out) that it has developed all the enzymes and mitochondria necessary to support this lifestyle.

You know you are keto-adapted when you: feel no hunger, feel no cravings for high-carb foods (your body is cured of the carbohydrate addiction), you have tons of energy, and you can sustain prolonged as well as high-intensity exercise with ease even in a fasted state.

You get into ketosis once your glycogen and glucose stores are depleted and your body starts shifting to using fat for energy driven purposes. Some people can get into ketosis in a couple of hours, while other people can do it in a couple of days.

Keto-adaptation starts occurring after a few weeks of constant ketosis and the process can be fully completed after a few months, sometimes after 1-2 years. This also depends on the fitness level of the individual, as Barry Murray relates.

6. Alternative Use for Coconut Oil

Besides cooking, I've heard people applying it to the skin, while other people applied it into their ears. We have learned that consuming coconut oil can be extremely helpful with conditions such as Alzheimer's Disease and other neurodegenerative diseases.

Some people use it in homemade deodorants and most of us use it as basis for our bulletproof coffee. Dr. Mercola [153] shows how coconut oil can be used as makeup remover, body scrub, facial scrub and cleanser, and even as shaving lotion. Some other uses are as: as toothpaste, as soap, as lip balm, and as insect repellant.

For medicinal purposes it can be used for: ear infections, bug bites, bee stings, skin irritations, skin rashes, cold sores, nosebleeds, and others [153]. See more at Dr. Mercola's website and try being inventive.

7. Normal Looking Meals

Some of you are saying that due to the high fat content and/or high fatty foods in this type of nutrition, the meals that you are eating would look odd. If you do not want to draw attention to your plate, just order some broccoli or kale with some steak and/or a glass of wine (if you must consume alcohol). Or you can order some eggs (omelet, scrambled, etc.) and order a salad with them.

I usually do not care what other people think. So far it's been vastly improved my health, fitness, productivity, and enhanced state of mind. That's what one should always consider when defending ketogenic nutrition.

8. How to tell people about your Way of Eating

To support what I've said earlier, I do not like to explain myself in front of others for my way of eating. But if you wish to share your experience about this, you should tell them that it is based on your research and experimentation. You will explain to them that high-fat-very-low-carb nutrition has a lot of benefits for health and fitness. What's more important is that you find it very enjoyable. It's just an honest appraisal of the truth.

You can always delve into the reference section of this book and find the studies that show the countless health benefits, such as:

protection against neurodegenerative diseases, protection against inflammation, as well as the unquestioned positive results with diabetes, epilepsy, obesity, and possibly in cancer. You can always go to Pub Med and/or Google Scholar and search for articles relating very-low-carb-high-fat nutrition and ketogenic diets.

The bottom line is that you don't have to be afraid to defend your position, even in front of your doctor. They may try to defend the high-carb dietary guidelines which are the established dogma. Show them that you are informed. If you breathe, eat, and look the same way you preach (i.e. if you show that ketogenic nutrition has helped you lose a lot of weight and become healthier) you will be more credible.

My doctor cannot believe how my lipid profile has improved while consuming big amounts of fat in the past couple of months.

9. Growth hormone and Ketosis

Some of you asked about the connection between growth hormone and ketosis. I would recommend reading one of the articles on my website which is entitled: Body Composition and Hormonal Changes under Low-Carb-High-Fat Nutrition.

I believe there is good correlation between the production of hormones and ketogenic diets because since there is a big supply of fat, the body is able to efficiently build hormones. You should know that most of the hormones in the body are made of fat and that cholesterol is the basic building block [154].

It is totally unwise to aim for lower cholesterol levels because you're depriving your body and your brain of one of the most important building blocks. Besides, cholesterol and phospholipids are found in the membranes of almost all of your body cells. Make sure you read Dr. Jack Kruse's blog to know more about this. His work is amazing.

10. High-Carb Meal Replacements and their High-Fat-Low-Carb Counter Parts

People can eat coconut flour pancakes and be happy they aren't depriving themselves of comfort food under ketogenic nutrition. The same strategies can be applied to find keto replacements for high-carb foods. Here are some of them. Again, I encourage you to be inventive and find your own substitutes:

normal pancakes - coconut, almond, or flax-seed flour pancakes

normal pizza - instead of regular wheat flour, again, try dough made with almond, coconut, or flax-seed flours.

Basically almost all high-carb wheat products can be replaced with the flours that I mentioned earlier. Sometimes it is difficult to find good low-carb products at the market, which is why I encourage you to do your own special keto foods.

mashed potatoes - mashed cauliflower (do a google search), mashed celery root

chocolate - dark chocolate

pasta - zucchini pasta or noodles, shirataki noodles

biscuits - coconut flour biscuits

cereals - flax-seed meal

french fries - fries made from swede, turnip, kohlrabi, parsley root, or even celery root

As you can see, good low-carb choices are only limited by your imagination. I encourage you to be inventive.

What about Supplements?

This is something of vital importance. I personally believe that one cannot get all the necessary vitamins and minerals from diet alone. Even if you have a well formulated very-low-carb-high-fat ketogenic diet [5], I would still choose to supplement.

Many critics of the ketogenic diet say that a diet where you have to use supplements is not good for you. But if you take a closer look at the general dietary guidelines, you can see they lack large amounts of vitamins and minerals. Where do you get your omega-3 fatty acids in the low fat high carb nutrition recommendation of the USDA? They only talk about vitamin D, folic acid, vitamin B12 and iron (for pregnant women) [155]. What about Potassium, Magnesium, Vitamin A, and others?

I am not here to write in a negative way about what others promote. I'm here to tell you about some of the evidence for supplements that served me well so far. These are also promoted by other big names in the low-carb arena.

One very important supplement that I use is **Alpha Lipoic Acid**. It is a very powerful anti-oxidant that fights the free radicals which result from the metabolism of food in your body. ALA is found in many foods but its concentration is extremely low. For example, one would have to eat a few tons of spinach to yield a few milligrams of ALA. That's why I advocate to using ALA supplements. I personally take 1 pill of ALA every day. The one that I use is made by a local pharma company and the product contains ALA+Biotin+Chromium. It's a combo that has been proven to work more efficiently when taken together.

The dosage of ALA that I take is 300mg. I'd have to eat a few dozen tons of spinach per day to get that amount from food. The biotin content is 300mcg, approximately 600% of the daily recommended intake. The chromium content is 200 mcg, approximately 500% of the daily recommended intake.

The next critically important supplement everyone should take is **omega-3 fatty acids**. The health benefits of this supplement are too numerous to list. You can do your own research on the Internet. I'd recommend that if you supplement with omega-3 fatty acids, make sure that it comes from reliable resources (that is cold water fish - and not laboratory grown fish).

I personally do not like to eat fish. I would have to consume a lot of fish every day just to get 1,000 mg of omega-3 that I get from 1 gelatin pill. The major health advantage of omega 3 fatty acids is that they are strongly anti-inflammatory.

I also take a **multi-vitamin and mineral pill** which contains the following:

Active Ingredient	Quantity	Daily Recommended %
Gingko Biloba Extract	50 mg	-
Lutein	500 µg	-
Vitamin A	800 µg	100%
Vitamin B1	1.1 mg	100%
Vitamin B2	1.4 mg	100%
Vitamin B6	1.4 mg	100%
Vitamin B12	2.5 µg	100%
Biotin	50 µg	100%
Folic Acid	200 µg	100%
Niacin	16 mg	100%
Pantothenic Acid	6 mg	100%
Vitamin C	80 mg	100%
Vitamin D3	5 µg	100%
Vitamin E	12 mg	100%
Vitamin K1	75 µg	100%
Calcium	120 mg	15%
Chromium	40 µg	100%
Iron	14 µg	100%
Fluoride	3.5 mg	100%
Iodine	150 µg	100%
Copper	1,000 µg	100%
Magnesium	56 mg	15%
Manganese	2 mg	100%
Molybdenum	50 µg	100%
Selenium	55 µg	100%
Zinc	10 mg	100%

All of these in the table above are found in one magic pill. You can see that I over-supplement (consume more than 100% of DRV) with some of the ingredients because I have chromium and biotin from my ALA pill too. However, I have not found this to have negative effects so far. I found no evidence, so far, that over-supplementation can be harmful.

You will notice that some of the ingredients do not provide 100% of the DRV such as Calcium and Magnesium. However, I get my Mg dose from the peanuts and other nuts that I consume daily. Other Mg rich foods are: leafy greens, dark chocolate and avocadoes. I then get my Ca daily dose through cheese, almonds, and dark leafy greens.

So far I've told you about **Alpha Lipoic Acid (+Biotin and Chromium), Omega 3 Fatty Acids, and Multi-Vitamin-Multi-Mineral pills.** But how much will this cost, you ask?

The 40 pills of ALA (+Biotin and Chromium) are $10. The stack lasts for 40 days. The Omega 3 Fatty Acid stack contains 30 pills and it costs $4. The Multi-Vitamin-Multi-Mineral (+Gingko and Lutein) pills come in a stack of 42 pills which costs $9. So the total cost for 1 month supply is ~$23. Your health and general well being is worth $23, is it not?

I also use something for the brain. It's called **CILTEP** and it promotes long-term potentiation. It improves memory and concentration and it boosts motivation. CILTEP is part of a new class of supplements called smart drugs and it's becoming more and more popular. I was one of the persons who tried this out as I was sent a sample stack by its producers. I found it to be very effective which is why I continued ordering it. You can find more information about CILTEP on one of the blog posts that I've written here [156]. You can order CILTEP here [157]. I want to emphasize that this is part of the optional supplements that I'm taking (and that it's not a daily necessity).

I also consume a teaspoon of **dried goji berries** along with my 85% cocoa dark chocolate every day. Goji berries are called the Chinese fountain of youth fruits because (same as ALA) they are powerful anti-oxidants and fight the free radicals (ROS - reactive oxygen species) in your body. If you decide to consume goji berries make sure they do not have preservatives and added sugars. Also, be aware that they are very high in carbohydrates (~70-80g of carbs per 100g of product). That's why I only consume a teaspoon of goji berries daily (which is approximately 2g of net carbs).

Other good supplements that I've tried are part of the **PAGG stack** promoted by Tim Ferriss in his book The 4 Hour Body [1]. PAGG as shown by Tim Ferriss and some of his followers seems to be working extremely well with his slow-carb diet (a type of low-carb diet) for the purpose of weight loss. PAGG stands for:

Policosanol (sugar cane extract)
Alpha Lipoic Acid
Garlic Extract
Green Tea Extract

I've taken each of these ingredients in the form of pills for up to 4 times a day. I didn't find it helped me lose weight on a 1 month slow-carb (6 days of moderately low carb + 1 day of carb loading) nutrition. However, I kept taking them as I started the ketogenic diet and I cannot say whether or not they contributed to the fat loss I experienced. Nevertheless, I believe in the effectiveness of each of these ingredients.

Green tea extract (decaffeinated) is very good for detoxification, higher energy levels, as well as weight-loss. Garlic extract is a powerful stimulant for the immune system and a detoxification agent, while policosanol is believed to be very effective in lowering blood sugar. You can find more about the PAGG stack and how to take it in Tim Ferriss' book [1].

Chapter Eight

My Virtual Academy

I write these last few words to express my immense gratitude to the people who inspired me to create this book. I want to emphasize that, besides my personal experiments, none of what is written in the book is the result of my pure thinking. Everything comes from experimentation, studies, and the observations of experts from various fields. You can read about each of these people's work and follow their studies to become more comprehensive in knowledge of human biochemistry, nutrition, health, and performance. So, without further ado:

Peter Attia - The Eating Academy - http://eatingacademy.com/

This video is what triggered my keto endeavor:

https://www.youtube.com/watch?v=NqwvcrA7oe8

Gary Taubes - Why we get Fat Discussion - https://www.youtube.com/watch?v=l59YyXpCT1M

It's one of the lectures I often watch.

Mark Sisson - Low Carb Paleo with Mark Sisson

https://www.youtube.com/watch?v=Um-a61rClSs

Khan Academy

Fat and Protein Metabolism Playlist -

https://www.youtube.com/playlist?list=PLbKSbFnKYVY0lFIZQsDo8ZfAq8oq8cgxg

Krebs Cycle and Oxidative Phosphorylation Playlist -

https://www.youtube.com/playlist?list=PLbKSbFnKYVY15SofrPeWQxBwq_Eg7BhKi

Endocrine System and Behavior Playlist -

https://www.youtube.com/playlist?list=PLbKSbFnKYVY1lsbBztAdGbhm4glK5vf3Q

The Endocrine System Playlist -

https://www.youtube.com/playlist?list=PLbKSbFnKYVY0Ql1Ki0M6CJPq8_Fm9E2cG

Overview of Metabolism Playlist -

https://www.youtube.com/playlist?list=PLbKSbFnKYVY24X0vW5FQn2YwHHUp1dlMW

Cell Membrane Overview Playlist -

https://www.youtube.com/playlist?list=PLbKSbFnKYVY3nhcxSp8RFFJK7p4Bur1Nj

Moof University

It includes in-depth and very comprehensive insight of metabolic processes. I often watch these lectures.

https://www.youtube.com/user/MoofUniversity

Ancestry Foundation

Great talks by experts on nutrition, health, and performance

https://www.youtube.com/user/AncestryFoundation

The IHMC

Same as The Ancestry Foundation. One of my favorite talks is Jeff Volek's https://www.youtube.com/watch?v=GC1vMBRFiwE

Jumpstart MD

https://www.youtube.com/user/JumpstartMD

One of my favorite interviews is the one with Steven Phinney and Jeff Volek:

https://www.youtube.com/watch?v=OFD2q5iqevY

Diet Doctor

Diet Doctor or Andreas Eenfeldt did various interviews with experts like: Robert Lustig, Gary Taubes, Peter Attia, Steven Phinney, Eric Westman, Mark Sisson, Loren Cordain and others.

https://www.youtube.com/user/eenfeldt

Dr. Mercola

I loved watching his interviews with Doug McGuff MD, Dr. Stephen Sinatra, and Dominic D'Agostino.

https://www.youtube.com/user/mercola

Kinesiology College

Great connection between metabolism and sports (kinetics). I loved these lectures because I find them very comprehensible.

https://www.youtube.com/user/KinesiologyCollege

All of these links as well as several other related articles, lectures, research studies, seminars, and debates, along with my personal experiments make up for the knowledge that I achieved in the field of nutrition, biochemistry, sports performance and health optimization. You can find more resources and some of the books I've read in the following reference section. I encourage you, the reader, not to take anything for granted. You should conduct your own research and apply the concepts in your life to determine what exactly works for you. There is no general prescription for anything. Even though our DNA is 99% the same, that 1% can make a hell of a difference. So I encourage you to adopt critical thinking and I really hope that this book will serve you as a reference for better nutrition, health, and performance.

Yours truly,
Cristi Vlad

References

1. Slow Carb Diet by Tim Ferriss - http://cristivlad.com/4hb

2. Peter Attia - An Advantaged Metabolic State: Human Performance, Resilience & Health - http://cristivlad.com/peter1

3. Aerobic - 8 minute Abs - http://cristivlad.com/eightminabs

4. The Ketogenic Experiment - http://cristivlad.com/ketoexperiment

5. Dr. Stephen Phinney and Dr. Jeff Volek - The Art and Science of Low-Carbohydrate Living - http://cristivlad.com/phinneyvolek

6. Aarsland, A., Chinkes, D., & Wolfe, R. R. (1997). Hepatic and whole-body fat synthesis in humans during carbohydrate overfeeding. *The American journal of clinical nutrition*, *65*(6), 1774-1782.

7. Diet Doctor – Why we get fat – with Gary Taubes http://cristivlad.com/gary1

8. Paoli, A., Grimaldi, K., D'Agostino, D., Cenci, L., Moro, T., Bianco, A., & Palma, A. (2012). Ketogenic diet does not affect strength performance in elite artistic gymnasts. *Journal of the International Society of Sports Nutrition*, *9*(1), 1-9.

9. Phinney, S. D., Bistrian, B. R., Evans, W. J., Gervino, E., & Blackburn, G. L. (1983). The human metabolic response to chronic ketosis without caloric restriction: preservation of submaximal exercise capability with reduced carbohydrate oxidation. *Metabolism*, *32*(8), 769-776.

10. Guzmán, M., & Blázquez, C. (2004). Ketone body synthesis in the brain: possible neuroprotective effects. *Prostaglandins, leukotrienes and essential fatty acids*, *70*(3), 287-292.

11. Morris, A. A. M. (2005). Cerebral ketone body metabolism. *Journal of inherited metabolic disease*, *28*(2), 109-121.

12. Ketostix (to measure urine ketones) - http://cristivlad.com/ketostix

13. Precision Xtra NFR Blood Glucose Monitoring System - http://cristivlad.com/bloodketones

14. Phinney, S. D. (2004). Ketogenic diets and physical performance. *Nutr Metab (Lond)*, *1*(1), 2.

15. McDonald, L. (1998). The Ketogenic Diet: A complete guide for the Dieter and Practitioner. Morris Publishing. - http://cristivlad.com/lyle

16. Gary Taubes - Good Calories, Bad Calories: Fat, Carbs, and the Controversial Science of Diet and Health - http://cristivlad.com/gary2

17. Westerterp - Plantenga, M. S., Lejeune, M. P., & Kovacs, E. M. (2005). Body weight loss and weight maintenance in relation to habitual caffeine intake and green tea supplementation. *Obesity research*, *13*(7), 1195-1204.

18. Psyllium Products - http://cristivlad.com/psyllium

19. Paoli, A., Bianco, A., Grimaldi, K. A., Lodi, A., & Bosco, G. (2013). Long Term Successful Weight Loss with a Combination Biphasic Ketogenic Mediterranean Diet and Mediterranean Diet Maintenance Protocol. *Nutrients*, *5*(12), 5205-5217.

20. Bueno, N. B., de Melo, I. S. V., de Oliveira, S. L., & da Rocha Ataide, T. (2013). Very-low-carbohydrate ketogenic diet v. low-fat diet for long-term weight loss: A meta-analysis of randomised controlled trials. *British Journal of Nutrition*, *110*(07), 1178-1187.

21. Partsalaki, I., Karvela, A., & Spiliotis, B. E. (2012). Metabolic impact of a ketogenic diet compared to a hypocaloric diet in obese children and adolescents. *Journal of Pediatric Endocrinology and Metabolism*, *25*(7-8), 697-704.

22. Beta-Oxidation - http://en.wikipedia.org/wiki/Beta_oxidation

23. U.F. Teaching Center - Beta Oxidation of Fatty Acids - http://cristivlad.com/ufbetaoxidation

24. Forsythe, C. E., Phinney, S. D., Fernandez, M. L., Quann, E. E., Wood, R. J., Bibus, D. M., ... & Volek, J. S. (2008). Comparison of low fat and low carbohydrate diets on circulating fatty acid composition and markers of inflammation. *Lipids*, *43*(1), 65-77.

25. Stubbs, R. J., Mazlan, N., & Whybrow, S. (2001). Carbohydrates, appetite and feeding behavior in humans. *The Journal of nutrition*, *131*(10), 2775S-2781S.

26. Milder, J., & Patel, M. (2012). Modulation of oxidative stress and mitochondrial function by the ketogenic diet. *Epilepsy research*, *100*(3), 295-303.

27. Klok, M. D., Jakobsdottir, S., & Drent, M. L. (2007). The role of leptin and ghrelin in the regulation of food intake and body weight in humans: a review. *Obesity reviews*, *8*(1), 21-34.

28. Sumithran, P., Prendergast, L. A., Delbridge, E., Purcell, K., Shulkes, A., Kriketos, A., & Proietto, J. (2013). Ketosis and appetite-mediating nutrients and hormones after weight loss. *European journal of clinical nutrition*, *67*(7), 759-764.

29. Goldberg, I. J., Eckel, R. H., & Abumrad, N. A. (2009). Regulation of fatty acid uptake into tissues: lipoprotein lipase-and CD36-mediated pathways. *Journal of lipid research*, *50*(Supplement), S86-S90.

30. Doug McGuff and John Little - Body by Science: A Research Based Program for Strength Training, Body building, and Complete Fitness in 12 Minutes a Week - http://cristivlad.com/bodybyscience

31. Wilcox, G. (2005). Insulin and insulin resistance. *Clinical Biochemist Reviews*, *26*(2), 19.

32. Denton RM, Tavaré JM. Molecular basis of insulin action on intracellular metabolism. In: Alberti KGMM, Zimmet P, Defronzo RA, Keen H (Hon), editors. International Textbook of Diabetes Mellitus (2nded) John Wiley & Sons, New York; 1997 p. 469–88.

33. American Diabetes Association (2014). Quick Breakfast Ideas - http://www.diabetes.org/food-and-fitness/food/what-can-i-eat/food-tips/quick-meal-ideas/quick-breakfast-ideas.html

34. Westman, E. C., Feinman, R. D., Mavropoulos, J. C., Vernon, M. C., Volek, J. S., Wortman, J. A., ... & Phinney, S. D. (2007). Low-carbohydrate nutrition and metabolism. *The American journal of clinical nutrition*, *86*(2), 276-284.

35. Volek, J. S., Phinney, S. D., Forsythe, C. E., Quann, E. E., Wood, R. J., Puglisi, M. J., ... & Feinman, R. D. (2009). Carbohydrate restriction has a more favorable impact on the metabolic syndrome than a low fat diet. *Lipids*, *44*(4), 297-309.

36. Westman, E. C., Yancy Jr, W. S., Mavropoulos, J. C., Marquart, M., & McDuffie, J. R. (2008). The effect of a low-carbohydrate, ketogenic diet versus a low-glycemic index diet on glycemic control in type 2 diabetes mellitus. *Nutr Metab (Lond)*, *5*, 36.

37. Yancy Jr, W. S., Foy, M., Chalecki, A. M., Vernon, M. C., & Westman, E. C. (2005). A low-carbohydrate, ketogenic diet to treat type 2 diabetes. *Nutr Metab (Lond)*, *2*, 34.

38. Dashti, H. M., Mathew, T. C., Khadada, M., Al-Mousawi, M., Talib, H., Asfar, S. K., & Al-Zaid, N. S. (2007). Beneficial effects of ketogenic diet in obese diabetic subjects. *Molecular and cellular biochemistry*, *302*(1-2), 249-256.

39. Center for Disease Control and Prevention (2011). Percentage of Civilian, Noninstitutionalized Population with Diagnosed Diabetes, by Age, United States, 1980 - 2011. Retrieved from http://www.cdc.gov/diabetes/statistics/prev/national/figbyage.htm

40. Center for Disease Control and Prevention (2012). Diabetes Report Card 2012: National and State Profile of Diabetes and Its Complications. Retrieved from http://www.cdc.gov/diabetes/pubs/reportcard/diabetes-incidence.htm

41. U.S. Department of Health and Human Services (n.d.). Scope of the Problem. Retrieved from http://aspe.hhs.gov/health/blueprint/scope.shtml

42. Ruge, T., Sukonina, V., Kroupa, O., Makoveichuk, E., Lundgren, M., Svensson, M. K., & Eriksson, J. W. (2012). Effects of hyperinsulinemia on lipoprotein lipase, angiopoietin-like protein 4, and glycosylphosphatidylinositol-anchored high-density lipoprotein binding protein 1 in subjects with and without type 2 diabetes mellitus. *Metabolism*, *61*(5), 652-660.

43. Kiens, B., Lithell, H., Mikines, K. J., & Richter, E. A. (1989). Effects of insulin and exercise on muscle lipoprotein lipase activity in man and its relation to insulin action. *Journal of Clinical Investigation*, *84*(4), 1124.

44. Jacobs, I., Lithell, H., & Karlsson, J. (1982). Dietary effects on glycogen and lipoprotein lipase activity in skeletal muscle in man. *Acta physiologica Scandinavica*, *115*(1), 85-90.

45. Peter Attia - The Eating Academy - Glossary - http://eatingacademy.com/glossary

46. Kulik-Rechberger, B. (2002). Leptin - The metabolic signal from adipose tissue. *Przeglad lekarski*, *60*(1), 35-39.

47. Dr. Jack Kruse (2011). Leptin: Chapter One. Retrieved from http://jackkruse.com/chapter-one-on-leptin/

48. Dr. Jack Kruse (2013). Epi-paleo Rx: The Prescription for Disease Reversal and Optimal Health - http://cristivlad.com/krusejack

49. Centers for Disease Control and Prevention (2012). Prevalence of Overweight, Obesity, and Extreme Obesity among Adults: United States, Trends 1960-1962 Through 2009-2010

50. Keys, A. (1980). Seven Countries: A Multivariate Analysis of Death and Coronary Heart Disease. Harvard University Press.

51. U.S. Government (1977). Dietary Goals for the United States (The McGovern Report).

52. Yerushalmy, J., & Hilleboe, H. E. (1957). Fat in the diet and mortality from heart disease; a methodologic note. *New York State journal of medicine*, *57*(14), 2343-2354.

53. Siri-Tarino, P. W., Sun, Q., Hu, F. B., & Krauss, R. M. (2010). Meta-analysis of prospective cohort studies evaluating the association of saturated fat with cardiovascular disease. *The American journal of clinical nutrition*, *91*(3), 535-546.

54. Roberts, R., Bickerton, A. S., Fielding, B. A., Blaak, E. E., Wagenmakers, A. J., Chong, M. F., ... & Frayn, K. N. (2008). Reduced oxidation of dietary fat after a short term high-carbohydrate diet. *The American journal of clinical nutrition*, *87*(4), 824-831.

55. Rosqvist, F., Iggman, D., Kullberg, J., Cedernaes, J. J., Johansson, H. E., Larsson, A., ... & Risérus, U. (2014). Overfeeding Polyunsaturated and Saturated Fat Causes Distinct Effects on Liver and Visceral Fat Accumulation in Humans. *Diabetes*, DB_131622.

56. National Institutes of Health (1988). The Reports of the Surgeon General. Retrieved from the National Library of Medicine: http://profiles.nlm.nih.gov/NN/B/C/Q/G/

57. Pennington, N. L. & Baker, C. W. (1990). Sugar: User's Guide to Sucrose. An Avi Book Series. - http://cristivlad.com/guidesucrose

58. Forsythe, C. E., Phinney, S. D., Feinman, R. D., Volk, B. M., Freidenreich, D., Quann, E., ... & Volek, J. S. (2010). Limited effect of dietary saturated fat on plasma saturated fat in the context of a low carbohydrate diet. *Lipids*, *45*(10), 947-962.

59. Gardner, C. D., Kiazand, A., Alhassan, S., Kim, S., Stafford, R. S., Balise, R. R., ... & King, A. C. (2007). Comparison of the Atkins, Zone, Ornish, and LEARN diets for change in weight and related risk factors among overweight premenopausal women: the A TO Z Weight Loss Study: a randomized trial. *Jama*, *297*(9), 969-977.

60. Biochemistry - Lipids and the Plasma Membrane. Retrieved from http://en.wikibooks.org/wiki/Biochemistry/Lipids_And_The_Plasma_Membrane

61. Chang, C. Y., Ke, D. S., & Chen, J. Y. (2009). Essential fatty acids and human brain. *Acta Neurol Taiwan*, *18*(4), 231-41.

62. Peter Attia - The Straight Dope on Cholesterol - Part I - Retrieved from http://eatingacademy.com/nutrition/the-straight-dope-on-cholesterol-part-i

63. Cristi Vlad - Privileged Metabolic State - 19.6% to 14.4% bodyfat in 2 Months [+Pics] - http://cristivlad.com/privileged

64. Lammert, F., & Wang, D. Q. H. (2005). New insights into the genetic regulation of intestinal cholesterol absorption. *Gastroenterology*, *129*(2), 718-734.

65. Lipoproteins, Apolipoproteins, and Familial Dyslipidemias Made Simple - http://cristivlad.com/lipoproteins

66. Stephen Sinatra and John Bowden - The Great Cholesterol Myth: Why Lowering Your Cholesterol Won't Prevent Heart Disease-and the Statin-Free Plan That Will - http://cristivlad.com/sinatra

67. Held, P. (2010). An Introduction to Reactive Oxygen Species. *BioTek White Paper*.

68. Addabbo, F., Montagnani, M., & Goligorsky, M. S. (2009). Mitochondria and reactive oxygen species. *Hypertension*, *53*(6), 885-892.

69. Eastern Kentucky University (2005). Human Physiology: Cell Structure and Function. Retrieved from http://people.eku.edu/ritchisong/301notes1.htm

70. Guyton, C. & Hall, J. E. (2010). *Medical Physiology*. Saunders. - http://cristivlad.com/guyton

71. King, M. W. (2014). Mitochondrial Functions and Biological Oxidations. Retrieved from http://themedicalbiochemistrypage.org/oxidative-phosphorylation.html#complexes

72. Murphy, M. (2009). How mitochondria produce reactive oxygen species. *Biochem. J, 417,* 1-13.

73. Haas, K., & Klingenspor, M. (2012). Age and high fat-diet associated changes in mitochondrial ROS production in the liver. *Biochimica et Biophysica Acta (BBA)-Bioenergetics, 1817,* S99.

74. Vial, G., Dubouchaud, H., Couturier, K., Cottet-Rousselle, C., Taleux, N., Athias, A., & Leverve, X. M. (2011). Effects of a high-fat diet on energy metabolism and ROS production in rat liver. *Journal of hepatology, 54*(2), 348-356.

75. Stafford, P., Abdelwahab, M. G., Kim, D. Y., Preul, M. C., Rho, J. M., & Scheck, A. C. (2010). The ketogenic diet reverses gene expression patterns and reduces reactive oxygen species levels when used as an adjuvant therapy for glioma. *Nutrition & metabolism, 7*(1), 74.

76. Maalouf, M., Sullivan, P. G., Davis, L., Kim, D. Y., & Rho, J. M. (2007). Ketones inhibit mitochondrial production of reactive oxygen species production following glutamate excitotoxicity by increasing NADH oxidation. *Neuroscience, 145*(1), 256-264.

77. Gregersen, S., Samocha-Bonet, D., Heilbronn, L. K., & Campbell, L. V. (2012). Inflammatory and oxidative stress responses to high-carbohydrate and high-fat meals in healthy humans. *Journal of nutrition and metabolism, 2012.*

78. Ratliff, J. C., Mutungi, G., Puglisi, M. J., Volek, J. S., & Fernandez, M. L. (2008). Eggs modulate the inflammatory response to carbohydrate restricted diets in overweight men. *Nutr Metab (Lond), 5*(1), 6.

79. Lorigados Pedre, L., ChacÃ³n, M., Lilia, M., Orozco, S., PavÃ³n Fuentes, N., Serrano, S. Ã., ... & Rocha Arrieta, L. (2013). Inflammatory mediators in epilepsy. *Current pharmaceutical design, 19*(38), 6766-6772.

80. Pagon, R. A., Adam, M. P., Bird, T. D., Dolan, C. R., Fong, C. T., & Stephens, K. (2014). Alzheimer Disease Overview--GeneReviews™.

81. Bianconi, E., Piovesan, A., Facchin, F., Beraudi, A., Casadei, R., Frabetti, F., & Canaider, S. (2013). An estimation of the number of cells in the human body. *Annals of human biology*, *40*(6), 463-471.

82. Shin, E. J., Jeong, J. H., Chung, Y. H., Kim, W. K., Ko, K. H., Bach, J. H., ... & Kim, H. C. (2011). Role of oxidative stress in epileptic seizures. *Neurochemistry international*, *59*(2), 122-137.

83. Yadav, A., Agrawal, S., Tiwari, S. K., & Chaturvedi, R. K. (2014). Mitochondria: Prospective Targets for Neuroprotection in Parkinson's Disease. *Current pharmaceutical design*.

84. Nuzzo, D., Picone, P., Caruana, L., Vasto, S., Barera, A., Caruso, C., & Di Carlo, M. (2013). Inflammatory Mediators as Biomarkers in Brain Disorders. *Inflammation*, 1-10.

85. Kossoff, E. (2011). Ketogenic Diets: Treatments for Epilepsy and Other Disorders - http://cristivlad.com/epilepsy

86. Mary Newport - Medium Chain Triglycerides and Ketones: An Alternative Fuel for Alzheimer's - http://www.youtube.com/watch?v=feyydeMFWy4

87. Vander Heiden, M. G., Cantley, L. C., & Thompson, C. B. (2009). Understanding the Warburg effect: the metabolic requirements of cell proliferation. *science*, *324*(5930), 1029-1033.

88. Marie, S. K. N., & Shinjo, S. M. O. (2011). Metabolism and brain cancer. *Clinics*, *66*, 33-43.

89. Van Kouwen, M. C. A., Oyen, W. J. G., Nagengast, F. M., Jansen, J. B. M. J., & Drenth, J. P. H. (2004). FDG-PET scanning in the diagnosis of gastrointestinal cancers. *Scandinavian Journal of Gastroenterology*, *39*(241), 85-92.

90. Dominic D'Agostino - Current and further researches - http://cristivlad.com/dominic

91. Thomas Seyfried - Cancer as a Metabolic Disease: On the Origin, Management, and Prevention of Cancer - http://cristivlad.com/seyfried

92. Arnal, M. A., Mosoni, L., Boirie, Y., Houlier, M. L., Morin, L., Verdier, E., & Mirand, P. P. (2000). Protein feeding pattern does not affect protein retention in young women. *The Journal of nutrition*, *130*(7), 1700-1704.

93. Soeters, M. R., Lammers, N. M., Dubbelhuis, P. F., Ackermans, M., Jonkers-Schuitema, C. F., Fliers, E., & Serlie, M. J. (2009). Intermittent fasting does not affect whole-body glucose, lipid, or protein metabolism. *The American journal of clinical nutrition*, *90*(5), 1244-1251.

94. Cleveland Clinic (2014). Calories Burned While Running. Retrieved from http://www.clevelandclinic.org/health/interactive/calories.asp

95. Ben Greenfield Blog (2013). The Great Ketogenic Ironman Experiment. Retrieved from http://www.bengreenfieldfitness.com/2013/05/low-carb-triathlon-training/

96. Jeff Volek (2013). The Many Facets of Keto-Adaptation. Retrieved from http://www.youtube.com/watch?v=GC1vMBRFiwE

97. Phinney, S. D., Bistrian, B. R., Evans, W. J., Gervino, E., & Blackburn, G. L. (1983). The human metabolic response to chronic ketosis without caloric restriction: preservation of submaximal exercise capability with reduced carbohydrate oxidation. *Metabolism*, *32*(8), 769-776.

98. Jeukendrup, A. E., & Aldred, S. (2004). Fat supplementation, health, and endurance performance. *Nutrition*, *20*(7), 678-688.

99. Ben Greenfield Blog (2013). The Ultimate Guide to Combining Fasting and Exercise: Everything you need to Know - Retrieved from http://www.bengreenfieldfitness.com/2014/02/combining-fasting-and-exercise/

100. Garcia-Roves, P., Huss, J. M., Han, D. H., Hancock, C. R., Iglesias-Gutierrez, E., Chen, M., & Holloszy, J. O. (2007). Raising plasma fatty acid concentration induces increased biogenesis of mitochondria in skeletal muscle. *Proceedings of the National Academy of Sciences*, *104*(25), 10709-10713.

101. Bough, K. J., Wetherington, J., Hassel, B., Pare, J. F., Gawryluk, J. W., Greene, J. G., ... & Dingledine, R. J. (2006). Mitochondrial biogenesis in the anticonvulsant mechanism of the ketogenic diet. *Annals of neurology*, *60*(2), 223-235.

102. Rho, J. M., & Rogawski, M. A. (2007). The Ketogenic Diet: Stoking the Powerhouse of the Cell. *Epilepsy Currents*, *7*(2), 58.

103. Ahola-Erkkilä, S., Carroll, C. J., Peltola-Mjösund, K., Tulkki, V., Mattila, I., Seppänen-Laakso, T., ... & Suomalainen, A. (2010). Ketogenic diet slows down mitochondrial myopathy progression in mice. *Human molecular genetics*, *19*(10), 1974-1984.

104. Bénit, P., & Rustin, P. (2012). Changing the diet to make more mitochondria and protect the heart. *Circulation research*, *110*(8), 1047-1048.

105. University of New Mexico (2014). Energy Systems. Retrieved from http://unm.edu

106. Oregon State University (2014). Storage Carbohydrate Metabolism. Retrieved from http://oregonstate.edu

107. Masaryk University (2014). Types of Muscle Fibers. Retrieved from http://www.fsps.muni.cz/

108. Schiaffino, S., & Reggiani, C. (2011). Fiber types in mammalian skeletal muscles. *Physiological reviews*, *91*(4), 1447-1531.

109. Mackenzie, B. (2014). Characteristics of Muscle Types. Retrieved from http://www.brianmac.co.uk/muscle.htm

110. Elmhurst College (2014). Glycogenesis, Glycogenolysis, and Gluconeogenesis. Retrieved from http://www.elmhurst.edu/~chm/vchembook/604glycogenesis.html

111. Sunny, N. E., & Bequette, B. J. (2011). Glycerol is a major substrate for glucose, glycogen, and nonessential amino acid synthesis in late-term chicken embryos. *Journal of animal science*, *89*(12), 3945-3953.

112. King, M. (2013). Gluconeogenesis: Glucose Synthesis. Retrieved from http://themedicalbiochemistrypage.org/gluconeogenesis.php

113. Manninen, A. H. (2006). Very-low-carbohydrate diets and preservation of muscle mass. *Nutr Metab (Lond)*, *3*(1), 9.

114. Jansson, E., Esbjörnsson, M., Holm, I., & Jacobs, I. (1990). Increase in the proportion of fast - twitch muscle fibres by sprint training in males. *Acta Physiologica Scandinavica*, *140*(3), 359-363.

115. Simoneau, J. A., Lortie, G., Boulay, M. R., Marcotte, M., Thibault, M. C., & Bouchard, C. (1985). Human skeletal muscle fiber type alteration with high-intensity intermittent training. *European journal of applied physiology and occupational physiology*, *54*(3), 250-253.

116. Nader, P. A. (2010). *Effects of short-term, high-force resistance training on high-intensity exercise capacity* (Doctoral dissertation, University of Louisville).

117. Häggmark, T., Eriksson, E., & Jansson, E. (1986). Muscle fiber type changes in human skeletal muscle after injuries and immobilization. *Orthopedics*, *9*(2), 181-185.

118. Ingjer, F. (1979). Effects of endurance training on muscle fibre ATP-ase activity, capillary supply and mitochondrial content in man. *The Journal of physiology*, *294*(1), 419-432.

119. Exercise Intelligence (2013). Are skeletal muscle fibers type in human fixed? Retrieved from http://www.exercise-intelligence.com/pdf/are%20skeletal%20muscle%20fibers%20fixed.pdf

120. Exercise and Leisure (2014). Commercial Strength Equipment. Retrieved from http://www.exerciseandleisure.com/

121. Cornell University (2014). Bicep Curls. Retrieved from http://blogs.cornell.edu/huang3040/files/2013/03/biceps-curl-2-pw1alb.png

122. PowerHouse Fitness (2014). BodyMax IT9301 Seated Chest Press Machine. Retrieved from http://www.powerhouse-fitness.co.uk/media/catalog/product/

123. Wikipedia (2014). Bench Press. Retrieved from http://upload.wikimedia.org/wikipedia/commons/thumb/b/b2/Bench-press.png/1024px-Bench-press.png

124. Worksquad (2014). Wide-Lat Pulldown and Close Grip Pulldown. Retrieved from http://workoutsquad.nl/

125. Organic Fitness (2014). Top 6 Exercises for a Muscular Physique. Retrieved from http://organicfitness.com/top-6-exercises-for-a-muscular-physique/

126. WorkoutLabs (2014). Bent Over Barbell Row. Retrieved from http://workoutlabs.com/exercise-guide/bent-over-barbell-row/

127. Nutriplanet (2014). Leg Press. Retrieved from http://www.nutriplanet.be/fitness-oefeningen.asp?training=Leg%20Press

128. Bodybuilding Monsters (2014). Mike Mentzer's High Intensity Training. Retrieved from https://www.youtube.com/watch?v=nZKbxtnJoq0

129. Hakkinen, K., Pakarinen, A., Alen, M., Kauhanen, H., & Komi, P. V. (1988). Neuromuscular and hormonal adaptations in athletes to strength training in two years. *Journal of Applied Physiology, 65*(6), 2406-2412.

130. Craig, B. W., Brown, R., & Everhart, J. (1989). Effects of progressive resistance training on growth hormone and testosterone levels in young and elderly subjects. *Mechanisms of ageing and development, 49*(2), 159-169.

131. Mercola, J. (2012). Super-Slow Weight Training: The Muscle Building Workout Hardly anyone Uses. Retrieved from http://fitness.mercola.com/sites/fitness/archive/2012/05/11/benefits-of-super-slow-workouts.aspx

132. Sato, K., Iemitsu, M., Matsutani, K., Kurihara, T., Hamaoka, T., & Fujita, S. (2014). Resistance training restores muscle sex steroid hormone steroidogenesis in older men. *The FASEB Journal*, fj-13.

133. Dr. Jack Kruse (2012). Cold Thermogenesis: The Ancient Pathway. Retrieved from http://jackkruse.com/cold-thermogenesis-6-the-ancient-pathway/

134. Silva, J. E. (2006). Thermogenic mechanisms and their hormonal regulation. *Physiological reviews*, *86*(2), 435-464.

135. Silva, J. E. (1995). Thyroid hormone control of thermogenesis and energy balance. *Thyroid*, *5*(6), 481-492.

136. Lowell, B. B., & Spiegelman, B. M. (2000). Towards a molecular understanding of adaptive thermogenesis. *Nature*, *404*(6778), 652-660.

137. Wikipedia (2014). Wim Hof, The Iceman. Retrieved from http://en.wikipedia.org/wiki/Wim_Hof

138. Daredevils (2013). The Ice Man. Retrieved from https://www.youtube.com/watch?v=6YcteEOu59c

139. Kox, M., Stoffels, M., Smeekens, S. P., van Alfen, N., Gomes, M., Eijsvogels, T. M., & Pickkers, P. (2012). The influence of concentration/meditation on autonomic nervous system activity and the innate immune response: a case study. *Psychosomatic medicine*, *74*(5), 489-494.

140. Lagakos, W. (2014). Fish, Dark Chocolate and Red Wine. Retrieved from http://caloriesproper.com/?p=4336

141. Lagakos, W. (2014). Going Dutch on Dark Chocolate. Retrieved from http://caloriesproper.com/?p=4266

142. Weinrich Chocolates (2014). Weinrich Black 85% Cocoa. Retrieved from http://www.weinrich-chocolates.com

143. Mercola, J. (2010). Coconut Oil: Four Tablespoons of this Brain Food May Prevent Alzheimer's. Retrieved from http://articles.mercola.com/sites/articles/archive/2010/12/13/can-this-natural-food-cure-or-prevent-alzheimers.aspx

144. Brads Greenhouse (2013). How to Crack Open a Fresh Coconut Quickly and Easily with Tools that Everybody Owns. Retrieved from https://www.youtube.com/watch?v=oFDePsAqxnI

145. Westman, E. C., Phinney, S. D. & Volek J. S. (2010). New Atkins for a New You: The Ultimate Diet for Shedding Weight and Feeling Great. - http://cristivlad.com/newatkins

146. Pinterest (2014). Keto Approved. Retrieved from http://www.pinterest.com/thatonekid/

147. Saumer, J. (2014). Keto-safe Foods. Retrieved from http://www.pinterest.com/jlsaumer/keto-safe-foods/

148. Ruled.me (2014). Keto Recipes. Retrieved from http://www.ruled.me/keto-recipes/

149. Ketodietapp (2014). Recipes. Retrieved from http://ketodietapp.com/Blog/category/Recipes

150. Bishop, M. (2014). Keto/Low-Carb. Retrieved from http://www.pinterest.com/heighyew/keto-low-carb/

151. Lewis, D. (n.d.). How to Keto. Retrieved from http://www.jones4fitness.com/resources/No_Sugar_No_Starch_Diet.doc

152. Gunnars, K. (2013). 4 Natural Sweeteners that are Good for Your Health. Retrieved from http://authoritynutrition.com/4-healthy-natural-sweeteners/

153. Mercola, J. (2013). Countless Uses for Coconut Oil - The Simple, the Strange, and the Downright Odd. Retrieved from http://articles.mercola.com/sites/articles/archive/2013/11/18/coconut-oil-uses.aspx

154. Mercola, J. (2000). Understanding Adrenal Function. Retrieved from http://articles.mercola.com/sites/articles/archive/2000/08/27/adrenals.aspx

155. U.S.D.A. (2010). Building Healthy Eating Patterns. Retrieved from http://www.cnpp.usda.gov/Publications/DietaryGuidelines/2010/PolicyDoc/Chapter5.pdf

156. Cristi Vlad (2014). Flow - The State of Perfect, Pure Happiness. Retrieved from http://cristivlad.com/flow-state-perfect-pure-happiness/

157. CILTEP - http://cristivlad.com/ciltep

Made in the USA
San Bernardino, CA
17 July 2014